P9-DWO-973

PROCEDURE CHECKLISTS FOR

FUNDAMENTALS OF

NURSING

THIRD EDITION

Judith M. Wilkinson, PhD, ARNP

Leslie S. Treas, PhD, RN, CPNP-PC, NNP-BC

Karen L. Barnett, DNP, RN

Mable H. Smith, BSN, MN, JD, PhD

 F.A. Davis Company • Philadelphia

F. A. Davis Company
1915 Arch Street
Philadelphia, PA 19103
www.fadavis.com

Copyright © 2016 by F. A. Davis Company

Copyright © 2007, 2011 by F. A. Davis Company. All rights reserved. This product is protected by copyright. No part of it may be reproduced, stored in a retrieval system, or transmitted in any form or by any means, electronic, mechanical, photocopying, recording, or otherwise, without written permission from the publisher.

Printed in the United States of America

Last digit indicates print number: 10 9 8 7 6 5 4 3 2 1

Publisher, Nursing: Lisa B. Houck
Director of Content Development: Darlene D. Pedersen
Senior Content Project Manager: Adrienne D. Simon
Content Project Manager: Christina L. Snyder
Special Projects Editor: Shirley A. Kuhn
Electronic Project Manager: Katherine E. Crowley
Design and Illustrations Manager: Carolyn O'Brien

As new scientific information becomes available through basic and clinical research, recommended treatments and drug therapies undergo changes. The author(s) and publisher have done everything possible to make this book accurate, up to date, and in accord with accepted standards at the time of publication. The author(s), editors, and publisher are not responsible for errors or omissions or for consequences from application of the book, and make no warranty, expressed or implied, in regard to the contents of the book. Any practice described in this book should be applied by the reader in accordance with professional standards of care used in regard to the unique circumstances that may apply in each situation. The reader is advised always to check product information (package inserts) for changes and new information regarding dose and contraindications before administering any drug. Caution is especially urged when using new or infrequently ordered drugs.

ISBN 13: 978-0-8036-4078-8

Authorization to photocopy items for internal or personal use, or the internal or personal use of specific clients, is granted by F. A. Davis Company for users registered with the Copyright Clearance Center (CCC) Transactional Reporting Service, provided that the fee of $.25 per copy is paid directly to CCC, 222 Rosewood Drive, Danvers, MA 01923. For those organizations that have been granted a photocopy license by CCC, a separate system of payment has been arranged. The fee code for users of the Transactional Reporting Service is: 978-0- 8036-4076-4/18 0 + $.25.

Introduction

These checklists are designed for teachers to use when evaluating student skills and for students to use when practicing skills or participating in peer check-offs. There are two types of checklist:
* For each procedure, a checklist containing all the procedural steps, created specifically for that procedure.
* One principles-based checklist that applies to all procedures.

The principles checklist can be used in two ways:
1. For evaluating students, especially in clinical settings, teachers can use it instead of the steps-based checklists. If you choose, you can evaluate all procedures using this one piece of paper. Simply make as many copies as you need. For example, if you have 8 students and you expect to evaluate 3 skills per day, then you will need 24 copies for a clinical day.
2. For all students, and for teachers who prefer the individual, steps-based forms, you should use the principles checklist as the first page for each of those. Make as many copies of the principles checklist as you need.

Contents

Chapter 23

Chapter 24

Chapter 25

Chapter 26

Chapter 37

Chapter 38

Chapter 39

PRINCIPLES-BASED CHECKLIST TO USE WITH ALL PROCEDURES

Procedure # _____ Procedure Title _____

Check (✓) S (Satisfactory) or NI (Needs Improvement)

PROCEDURE STEPS	S	NI	COMMENTS
Before Approaching Patient:			
• Checks records (e.g., medication record) or obtains a prescription, if necessary. • Refers to agency protocols, if not familiar with them. • Obtains signed informed consent, if needed. • Performs hand hygiene; dons procedure gloves, if needed. • Gathers supplies and equipment before approaching patient. • Obtains assistance, if needed (e.g., to move a patient).			
Preparing Patient:			
• Introduces self and instructor to patient. • Identifies patient: reads wrist band, and asks patient to state his name. Follows agency protocol. • Makes relevant assessments (e.g., takes vital signs) to ensure that patient still requires the procedure, is able to tolerate it, and that there are no contraindications. • Explains the procedure to patient, including what he will feel and need to do (e.g., "You will need to lie very still"). • Provides privacy (e.g., asks visitors to step out, drapes patient). Uses good body mechanics: positions bed or treatment table to a working level; lowers the near siderail. • Uses good body mechanics: positions bed or treatment table to a working level; lowers the near siderail.			
During the Procedure:			
• Performs hand hygiene before touching patient, before gloving, after removing gloves, and again before leaving the room. • Observes universal precautions (e.g., dons and changes procedure gloves when needed). • Maintains sterility when needed. • Maintains correct body mechanics. • Provides patient safety (e.g., keeps siderail up on far side of the bed). • Continues to observe patient while performing the procedure steps and pauses or stops the procedure if patient is not tolerating it. • Performs the procedure within an acceptable time period.			

Copyright © 2016, F. A. Davis Company, Wilkinson & Treas/Procedure Checklists for Fundamentals of Nursing, 3e

PROCEDURE STEPS	S	NI	COMMENTS
• Demonstrates coordination in handling equipment. • Follows correct procedure steps.			
After the Procedure: • Evaluates patient's response to the procedure. • Leaves patient in a comfortable, safe position with the call light within reach. • If patient is in bed, returns the bed to the low position and raises the siderail (if patient requires this precaution). • Disposes of supplies and materials according to agency policy. • Washes hands again before leaving the room. • Documents that the procedure was done; documents patient's responses.			

Note: All procedures are "rules of thumb." Everything you learn can be altered by medical prescriptions, new information, agency policies, and individual patient needs. Every procedure requires nursing judgment.

Recommendation: Pass _____ Needs more practice _____

Student: _____   Date: _____

Instructor: _____   Date: _____

2   Copyright © 2016, F. A. Davis Company, Wilkinson & Treas/Procedure Checklists for Fundamentals of Nursing, 3e

PROCEDURE CHECKLIST
Chapter 9: Assessing for Abuse

Check (✓) Yes or No

PROCEDURE STEPS	Yes	No	COMMENTS
Before, during, and after the procedure, follows Principles-Based Checklist to Use With All Procedures, including: Identifies the patient according to agency policy; attends appropriately to standard precautions, hand hygiene, safety, privacy, and body mechanics.			
1. Assesses for abuse any time a child or dependent person has an injury.			
2. Uses a nonjudgmental approach.			
3. Does not make assumptions.			
4. Determines whether the injury was intentional or accidental.			
5. Obtains a focused health history, including assessing for physical, sexual, and psychological abuse or neglect.			
a. Questions patient and caregivers separately.			
b. Compares behavior to developmental level.			
c. Asks about past injuries or incidents.			
d. Asks detailed questions about how and when the injury occurred.			
e. Asks about inappropriate touching.			
f. Asks about genitourinary symptoms and vaginal discharge.			
g. Obtains data about aggressive or self-destructive behaviors (e.g., substance abuse).			
h. As appropriate, asks if victim is pregnant.			
i. Assesses for psychological abuse.			
j. Obtains information about who manages the family finances.			
6. Determines whether the caregiver has a history of a mental health disorder or substance abuse.			
7. Performs a focused physical assessment.			
a. Assesses present injury; looks for evidence of previous injuries.			
b. Notes cues such as bruises in the outline of a hand or cord loop, burns to feet and lower legs, circular burns, bite marks, injuries in the "triangle of safety" and the "swimsuit zone."			

PROCEDURE STEPS	Yes	No	COMMENTS
c. Assesses for bleeding or bruising of genitalia, poor sphincter tone, encopresis, and bruises on inner thighs.			
d. Observes for signs of neglect, such as poor hygiene, malnutrition, matted hair, clothing inappropriate for the weather.			
8. Ensures the integrity of evidence that may be needed for criminal prosecution.			
9. For any sexual examination, has a witness in the room, a SANE if possible.			
10. Assesses whether the injuries are consistent with the history.			
11. As appropriate, provides the victim with referrals for help in escaping the abusive situation.			
12. If appropriate, refers the parent, caregiver, or partner involved in the abuse to hotlines or agencies focused on stopping the abuse and protecting the victim.			
13. Reports abuse according to agency, state, and federal guidelines.			
14. Treats physical injuries or refers to the primary care provider for medical care.			

Recommendation: Pass _____ Needs more practice _____

Student: _____   Date: _____

Instructor: _____   Date: _____

    Copyright © 2016, F. A. Davis Company, Wilkinson & Treas/Procedure Checklists for Fundamentals of Nursing, 3e

PROCEDURE CHECKLIST
Chapter 11: Admitting a Patient to a Nursing Unit

Check (✔) Yes or No

PROCEDURE STEPS	Yes	No	COMMENTS
Before, during, and after the procedure, follows Principles-Based Checklist to Use With All Procedures, including: Identifies the patient according to agency policy; attends appropriately to standard precautions, hand hygiene, safety, privacy, and body mechanics.			
1. Introduces self to patient and family.			
2. Assists patient into a hospital gown.			
3. Measures weight, with patient standing on a scale if possible.			
4. Transfers or assists patient into the bed.			
5. Checks patient's identification band to ensure information, including allergies, is correct. Verifies this information with patient or family.			
6. Measures patient's vital signs.			
7. Completes nursing admission assessment (including health history) and physical assessment.			
8. Checks the list of the patient's current medications (created in the Admitting Department) for accuracy.			
9. Orients the patient to the room: Explains equipment, including how to use the call system, and the location of personal care items.			
10. Explains hospital routines, including use of siderails, mealtimes, and so on, and answers patient's and family's questions.			
11. Verifies with patient that all admission data on the chart are complete and correct.			
12. Asks if patient has an advance directive.			
13. Advises patient of privacy rights under the Health Insurance Portability and Accountability Act (HIPAA), with written explanation.			
14. Completes inventory of patient's belongings. Encourages the family to take home valuable items. If that is not possible, arranges to have valuables placed in the hospital safe.			
15. Ensures that all admission orders have been completed.			
16. Ensures patient comfort (e.g., positioning, water pitcher).			
17. Makes one last safety check (e.g., call light in reach, bed in low position, equipment functioning properly).			

Copyright © 2016, F. A. Davis Company, Wilkinson & Treas/Procedure Checklists for Fundamentals of Nursing, 3e

PROCEDURE STEPS	Yes	No	COMMENTS
18. Before leaving, asks if the nurse can do anything else for the patient or family.			
19. Initiates care plan or clinical pathway.			
20. Documents all findings.			

<u>Recommendation</u>: Pass _____ Needs more practice _____

Student: _____   Date: _____

Instructor: _____   Date: _____

PROCEDURE CHECKLIST
Chapter 11: Discharging a Patient From a Nursing Unit

Check (✔) Yes or No

PROCEDURE STEPS	Yes	No	COMMENTS
Before, during, and after the procedure, follows Principles-Based Checklist to Use With All Procedures, including: Identifies the patient according to agency policy; attends appropriately to standard precautions, hand hygiene, safety, privacy, and body mechanics.			
1. Notifies patient/family well in advance of discharge.			
2. About 48 hours before discharge: a. Arranges or confirms transportation, services, and equipment patient will need at home.			
b. Makes referrals.			
c. Provides teaching and training (condition and use of equipment).			
d. Asks the caregiver to bring patient's clothing, if needed.			
3. Day of discharge: a. Makes and documents final assessments.			
b. Confirms that patient has house keys, heat is turned on, and food is available at home.			
c. Makes final notifications (e.g., home care, transportation).			
d. Gives prescriptions, instruction sheets, and appointment cards to patient.			
e. Packs personal items and treatment supplies.			
f. Labels and packs medications.			
g. Documents final note; completes discharge summary.			
h. Reviews discharge summary with patient; provides printed copy; answers questions and addresses concerns.			
i. Accompanies patient out of the hospital.			

PROCEDURE STEPS	Yes	No	COMMENTS
j. Notifies Admissions of the discharge.			
k. Ensures records are sent to medical records department.			

Recommendation: Pass _____ Needs more practice _____

Student: _____   Date: _____

Instructor: _____   Date: _____

 Copyright © 2016, F. A. Davis Company, Wilkinson & Treas/Procedure Checklists for Fundamentals of Nursing, 3e

PROCEDURE CHECKLIST

Chapter 11: Transferring a Patient to Another Unit in the Agency

Check (✔) Yes or No

PROCEDURE STEPS	Yes	No	COMMENTS
Before, during, and after the procedure, follows Principles-Based Checklist to Use With All Procedures, including: Identifies the patient according to agency policy; attends appropriately to standard precautions, hand hygiene, safety, privacy, and body mechanics.			
1. Explains transfer to patient ahead of time, if possible.			
2. Obtains enough assistance to ensure safe transfer.			
3. Gathers and labels medications for the new room.			
4. Notifies the receiving unit and other departments (e.g., Dietary, Admitting).			
5. Brings a utility cart to the room if it is needed to transport patient's supplies and personal belongings.			
6. Places patient's personal belongings in a container for transfer.			
7. Brings a wheelchair or stretcher to bedside; assists patient to the wheelchair or stretcher.			
8. If patient must be transferred with equipment running (e.g., portable oxygen), obtains it ahead of time and sets it up for the transfer.			
9. Takes patient to the new room.			
10. Gives the handoff report, including all items on the structured format, or: name, age, physicians, surgical procedures and medical diagnoses, allergies, lab data, special equipment, current health status, status of advance directives and CPR, nursing diagnoses, and priorities for nursing care.			
11. Documents per agency policies.			

Recommendation: Pass _____ Needs more practice _____

Student: _____   Date: _____

Instructor: _____   Date: _____

Copyright © 2016, F. A. Davis Company, Wilkinson & Treas/Procedure Checklists for Fundamentals of Nursing, 3e

PROCEDURE CHECKLIST
Chapter 11: Transferring a Patient to a Long-Term Care Facility

Check (✓) Yes or No

PROCEDURE STEPS	Yes	No	COMMENTS
Before, during, and after the procedure, follows Principles-Based Checklist to Use With All Procedures, including: Identifies the patient according to agency policy; attends appropriately to standard precautions, hand hygiene, safety, privacy, and body mechanics.			
1. Notifies patient/family well in advance of transfer.			
2. Prepares and copies patient records for the receiving facility.			
3. Packs patient's personal items for transfer.			
4. Arranges for transportation.			
5. Checks medications for correct labeling; prepares them for transfer, as appropriate.			
6. Assists patient into a hospital gown.			
7. Notifies the receiving facility of transfer time and special equipment patient will need.			
8. Notifies Admitting, other hospital departments, physician, and family of the transfer; confirms transportation.			
9. Just before transfer, makes final assessment and signs off charting.			
10. When transportation arrives, takes patient to the vehicle; or hands off patient to transporters in patient's room. Removes patient's identification band per agency policy.			

11. Gives an oral report to long-term care facility nurse that includes:
    a. Reason for transfer
    b. Physical and psychosocial status
    c. Summary of care, treatment provided, and progress toward outcomes
    c. Referrals and community resources provided to patient			

12. Notifies receiving facility if patient is colonized or infected with methicillin-resistant *Staphylococcus aureus* (MRSA) or other contagious microorganisms.			

PROCEDURE STEPS	Yes	No	COMMENTS
13. If patient has an IV, oxygen, or equipment that cannot be turned off for transfer, notifies the receiving agency far enough in advance so that the agency can make it available.			

Recommendation: Pass _____ Needs more practice _____

Student: _____   Date: _____

Instructor: _____   Date: _____

PROCEDURE CHECKLIST
Chapter 20: Assessing the Apical Pulse

Check (✓) Yes or No

PROCEDURE STEPS	Yes	No	COMMENTS
Before, during, and after the procedure, follows Principles-Based Checklist to Use With All Procedures, including: Identifies the patient according to agency policy; attends appropriately to standard precautions, hand hygiene, safety, privacy, body mechanics, and documentation.			
1. Assists patient to a supine or sitting position (preferably sitting); exposes left side of the chest, only as much as necessary.			
2. Cleans the stethoscope with a 70% alcohol or benzalkonium chloride wipe before using.			
3. Selects, correctly locates, and palpates the apical site (5th intercostal space at the midclavicular line).			
4. Warms the stethoscope in the hands for 10 seconds.			
5. Uses the diaphragm of stethoscope over the PMI.			
6. Counts for 60 seconds.			
7. Notes rate, rhythm, and quality.			
8. Identifies S_1 and S_2 heart sounds.			
9. Again cleans the stethoscope with a 70% alcohol or benzalkonium chloride wipe.			

Recommendation: Pass _____ Needs more practice _____

Student: _____   Date: _____

Instructor: _____   Date: _____

Chapter 20: Assessing for an Apical–Radial Pulse Deficit

Check (✓) Yes or No

PROCEDURE STEPS	Yes	No	COMMENTS
Before, during, and after the procedure, follows Principles-Based Checklist to Use With All Procedures, including: Identifies the patient according to agency policy; attends appropriately to standard precautions, hand hygiene, safety, privacy, body mechanics, and documentation.			
1. Cleans the stethoscope before examining patient.			
2. Obtains another nurse to assist.			
3. Exposes left side of patient's chest, minimizing exposure.			
4. Places the watch so the second hand is visible to both nurses.			
5. Nurse 1 correctly locates and palpates the apical site (5th intercostal space at the midclavicular line) and uses diaphragm of stethoscope to auscultate the apex.			
6. Nurse 2 palpates the radial pulse and assesses rate, rhythm, and quality; correctly locates sites.			
7. Nurse 2 calls "start" to begin counting and "stop" to end the count.			
8. Counts for 60 seconds.			
9. Identifies S_1 and S_2 heart sounds.			
10. Correctly obtains pulse deficit (apical rate minus radial rate).			
Variation: When performing this procedure without a second nurse to assist, holds the stethoscope in place with one hand while palpating the radial pulse with the hand wearing the watch. If it is not possible to count both rates, at least report whether there are any differences between the apical and radial rates.			

Recommendation: Pass _____ Needs more practice _____

Student: _____   Date: _____

Instructor: _____   Date: _____

PROCEDURE CHECKLIST
Chapter 20: Assessing Body Temperature

Check (✓) Yes or No

PROCEDURE STEPS	Yes	No	COMMENTS
Before, during, and after the procedure, follows Principles-Based Checklist to Use With All Procedures, including: Identifies the patient according to agency policy; attends appropriately to standard precautions, hand hygiene, safety, privacy, body mechanics, and documentation.			
1. Cleans thermometer before and after use if it is not disposable.			
2. Selects the appropriate site and thermometer type.			
3. "Zeroes" or shakes down glass or plastic thermometers to 96°F (36°C) as needed.*			
4. Inserts the thermometer in a protective sheath or uses a thermometer designated only for patient.			
5. Inserts in chosen route/site. a. *Axillary*: Dries axilla; places the thermometer tip in the middle of the axilla; lowers patient's arm.			
b. *Oral*: Places the thermometer tip under the tongue in the posterior sublingual pocket (right or left of frenulum). Asks patient to keep lips closed.			
c. *Rectal*: Slides thermometer into a protective sheath; assists patient to Sims' position; uses rectal thermometer; lubricates thermometer; dons procedure gloves; inserts 2.5–3.7 cm (1–1.5 in.) in an adult; 2.5 cm (0.9 in.) for a child, and 1.5 cm (0.5 in.) for an infant. Holds thermometer securely in place; does not leave patient unattended.			
d. *Temporal Artery Temperature:* Removes the protective cap; cleans the lens/probe; places probe flat on center of the forehead; presses and holds button while stroking thermometer medially to laterally across the forehead; still holding the button, touches thermometer lens/probe behind the ear lobe; releases button to read temperature.			

PROCEDURE STEPS	Yes	No	COMMENTS
e. *Tympanic membrane*: Assures that thermometer lens is intact and clean; places disposable cover smoothly over the lens; positions patient's head to one side and straightens the ear canal. Unless manufacturer directs otherwise: 1) For an adult, pulls the pinna up and back. 2) For a child, pulls the pinna down and back. Inserts the probe in the ear canal and rotates it toward the jaw.			
f. *Skin Temperature, Chemical Strip Thermometer:* Places strip on the patient's skin; leaves in place 15 to 60 seconds; observes for color changes; reads temperature before removing strip from the skin; discards the thermometer strip.			
6. Leaves a glass or plastic thermometer for the recommended time (oral 5–8 minutes, rectal 3–5 minutes, axillary 8 minutes).			
7. Leaves an electronic thermometer until it beeps.			
8. Reads the temperature. (For a glass or plastic thermometer, wipes with tissue before reading; reads at eye level.)			
9. Shakes down (glass or plastic thermometer) and cleans it.			
10. Stores in recharging unit (electronic) or safe container (for glass or plastic).			

*Mercury-containing thermometers are not recommended. Use only glass or plastic thermometers filled with galinstan or alcohol.

Recommendation: Pass _____ Needs more practice _____

Student: _____   Date: _____

Instructor: _____   Date: _____

PROCEDURE CHECKLIST
Chapter 20: Assessing Peripheral Pulses

Check (✓) Yes or No

PROCEDURE STEPS	Yes	No	COMMENTS
NOTE: You can use this checklist to evaluate one peripheral pulse, or to evaluate the student's ability to locate all the peripheral pulses.			
Before, during, and after the procedure, follows Principles-Based Checklist to Use With All Procedures, including: Identifies the patient according to agency policy; attends appropriately to standard precautions, hand hygiene, safety, privacy, body mechanics, and documentation.			

Circle the site used:
    radial, brachial, carotid, dorsalis pedis, femoral,
    popliteal, posterior tibial, temporal			

1. Selects, correctly locates, and palpates the site.			
2. Uses fingers (not thumb) to palpate.			
3. Counts for 30 seconds if regular; 60 seconds if irregular.			
4. Notes rate, rhythm, and quality.			
5. Compares bilaterally.			
6. Carotid pulse: Palpates only on one side at a time.			
7. Correctly locates the following sites: a. Radial			
b. Brachial			
c. Carotid			
d. Dorsalis pedis			
e. Femoral			
f. Posterior tibial			
g. Popliteal			
h. Temporal			

Recommendation: Pass _____ Needs more practice _____

Student: _____   Date: _____

Instructor: _____   Date: _____

PROCEDURE CHECKLIST
Chapter 20: Assessing Respirations

Check (✓) Yes or No

PROCEDURE STEPS	Yes	No	COMMENTS
Before, during, and after the procedure, follows Principles-Based Checklist to Use With All Procedures, including: Identifies the patient according to agency policy; attends appropriately to standard precautions, hand hygiene, safety, privacy, body mechanics, and documentation.			
1. Positions the patient sitting or in Fowler's position, if possible.			
2. Flexes patient's arm and places patient's forearm across his chest, or otherwise counts unobtrusively.			
3. Palpates and counts the radial pulse, remembering the number.			
4. Keeping fingers on the patient's wrist, counts respirations.			
5. Observes rate, rhythm, and depth.			
6. Counts the number of breaths for 30 seconds if respirations are regular; 60 seconds if irregular. Begins timing with a count of 1 (if queried).			

Recommendation: Pass _____ Needs more practice _____

Student: _____   Date: _____

Instructor: _____   Date: _____

PROCEDURE CHECKLIST
Chapter 20: Measuring Blood Pressure (Brachial Artery)

Check (✓) Yes or No

PROCEDURE STEPS	Yes	No	COMMENTS
NOTE: This checklist describes using the brachial artery in the upper arm; however, the checklist can also be used to assess lower arm, calf, and thigh blood pressures.			
Before, during, and after the procedure, follows Principles-Based Checklist to Use With All Procedures, including: Identifies the patient according to agency policy; attends appropriately to standard precautions, hand hygiene, safety, privacy, body mechanics, and documentation.			
1. Cleans the stethoscope before beginning the procedure.			
2. Measures blood pressure after patient has been inactive for 5 minutes.			
3. If possible, positions patient sitting, feet on floor, legs uncrossed; alternatively, lying down.			
4. Exposes an arm (does not auscultate through clothing).			
5. Supports patient's arm at the level of the heart.			
6. Uses appropriately sized cuff. (The width of the bladder of a properly fitting cuff will cover approximately ⅔ of the length of the upper arm for an adult, and the entire upper arm for a child. Alternatively, the length of the bladder encircles 80% to 100% of the arm in adults.)			
7. Positions the cuff correctly; wraps snugly; ensures it is totally deflated.			
8. Places stethoscope earpieces in own ears.			
9. Palpates the brachial artery on cuff arm: a. Closes the sphygmomanometer valve.			
b. Inflates the cuff rapidly to about 80 mm Hg.			
c. While palpating the pulse, continues inflating in 10 mm Hg increments until the pulse is no longer felt.			
d. Notes the pressure at which the pulse disappears.			
e. Continues inflating for 20–30 mm Hg more. f. Moves to Step 11.			

PROCEDURE STEPS	Yes	No	COMMENTS
10. **Variations in Cuff Inflation (step 9).** Palpates the brachial artery: a. Closes the sphygmomanometer valve.			
b. Inflates the cuff rapidly to about 80 mm Hg.			
c. While palpating the pulse, continues inflating in 10 mm Hg increments until the pulse is no longer felt.			
d. Notes the pressure at which the pulse disappears.			
e. Deflates the cuff rapidly.			
f. Waits 2 minutes, then places the stethoscope over the brachial artery and inflates the cuff to a pressure that is 20–30 mm Hg above the level previously palpated. Moves to Step 11.			
11. Places the stethoscope over the brachial artery, ensuring that: a. The stethoscope is not touching anything (e.g., clothing).			
b. The diaphragm is not tucked under the edge of the blood pressure cuff.			
12. Releases pressure at 2–3 mm Hg/second.			
13. Records at least systolic and diastolic readings (first and last sounds heard—e.g., 110/80). Records level of muffling, if possible.			
14. If necessary to remeasure, deflates cuff completely and waits at least 2 minutes.			
14. **Variation.** If a mercury manometer must be used, reads the scale at eye level.			
15. **Variation. If an automatic blood pressure device is used:** a. Follows the same guidelines as for taking a manual blood pressure (e.g., cuff size and placement, patient position).			
b. Turns on the machine, making sure the cuff is deflated.			
c. Applies the cuff; presses the button to start the measurement.			
d. At the tone, reads the digital measurement.			

 Copyright © 2016, F. A. Davis Company, Wilkinson & Treas/Procedure Checklists for Fundamentals of Nursing, 3e

PROCEDURE STEPS	Yes	No	COMMENTS
Procedure Variation A. Measuring Blood Pressure in the Forearm			
1. Uses properly sized cuff for forearm; places midway between the elbow and the wrist			
2. Uses above procedure, but auscultates over radial artery.			
3. Correctly locates radial artery.			
Procedure Variation B. Measuring Blood Pressure in the Thigh			
1. Places the patient in a prone position; alternatively, supine with knee slightly bent.			
2. Uses the correct cuff size; wraps the cuff so lower edge is 1 in. above the popliteal fossa and centered over the popliteal artery.			
3. Auscultates and palpates over the popliteal artery.			
Procedure Variation C. Measuring Blood Pressure in the Calf			
1. Places the patient in a supine position.			
2. Uses the correct cuff size; wraps the cuff so the lower edge is 1 in. above the malleoli or ankle.			
3. Places the stethoscope over the dorsalis pedis or the posterior tibial artery.			
Procedure Variation D. Palpating the Blood Pressure			
1. Applies the cuff, and palpates for the radial or brachial pulse.			
2. Inflates the cuff until the pulse disappears, then inflates for 30 mm Hg more.			
3. Releases the valve, slowly deflating the pulse.			
4. Notes manometer reading when pulse was felt again and records palpated reading.			

Recommendation: Pass _____ Needs more practice _____

Student: _____   Date: _____

Instructor: _____   Date: _____

Copyright © 2016, F. A. Davis Company, Wilkinson & Treas/Procedure Checklists for Fundamentals of Nursing, 3e

PROCEDURE CHECKLIST
Chapter 22: Assessing the Abdomen

Check (✔) Yes or No

PROCEDURE STEPS	Yes	No	COMMENTS
Before, during, and after the procedure, follows Principles-Based Checklist to Use With All Procedures, including: Identifies patient using two identifiers and according to agency policy; attends appropriately to standard precautions, hand hygiene, safety, privacy, and body mechanics.			
1. Has the client void prior to the exam.			
2. Positions the client supine with the knees slightly flexed.			
3. Examines abdomen in this order: inspection, auscultation, percussion, palpation.			
4. Inspects the abdomen for:			
a. Size, symmetry, and contour.			
b. Has client raise his head to check for bulges.			
c. If distention is present, measures girth at umbilicus with tape measure.			
d. Observes the condition of skin and skin color; lesions, scars, striae, superficial veins, and hair distribution.			
e. Notes abdominal movements.			
f. Notes position, contour, and color of the umbilicus.			
5. Auscultates the abdomen for bowel sounds, using diaphragm of stethoscope.			
a. Listens for up to 5 min. before concluding that bowel sounds are absent.			
b. Uses stethoscope bell to listen for bruits.			
c. Listens for bruits over aorta and renal, femoral, and iliac arteries.			
5a. Uses indirect percussion to assess at multiple sites in all four quadrants.			
5b. Estimates size of liver, spleen, and bladder.			
6. Uses fist or blunt percussion to percuss the costovertebral angle for tenderness.			
7. Palpates abdomen:			
a. Palpates in an organized manner. Begins with light palpation then uses deep palpation to palpate organs and masses.			
b. For light palpation, presses down 1–2 cm in a rotating motion. Identifies surface characteristics, tenderness, muscular resistance, and turgor.			

PROCEDURE STEPS	Yes	No	COMMENTS

8. Palpates liver:
   a. Stands on client's right side.
   b. Places right hand at the client's midclavicular line under and parallel to the costal margin.			

c. Places left hand under the client's back at the lower ribs and pressing upward.			
d. Asks client to inhale and deeply exhale while pressing in and up with the right fingers.			
9. Palpates spleen: a. Stands at client's right side.			
b. Places left hand under costovertebral angle and pulls upward.			
c. Places right hand under the left costal margin.			
d. Asks client to exhale and presses hands inward to palpate spleen.			

Recommendation: Pass _____ Needs more practice _____

Student: _____   Date: _____

Instructor: _____   Date: _____

Chapter 22: Assessing the Anus and Rectum

Check (✓) Yes or No

PROCEDURE STEPS	Yes	No	COMMENTS
Before, during, and after the procedure, follows Principles-Based Checklist to Use With All Procedures, including: Identifies patient using two identifiers and according to agency policy; attends appropriately to standard precautions, hand hygiene, safety, privacy, and body mechanics.			
1. Inspects the anus: skin noting condition, lesions.			

2. Palpates the anus and rectum.
   a. *For women*: Changes gloves to prevent cross-contamination. Inserts a lubricated index finger gently into the rectum. Palpates the rectal wall noting masses or tenderness.
   b. *For men*: Has the client bend over the exam table or turn on his left side if recumbent. Inserts a lubricated, gloved index finger gently into the rectum. Palpates the rectal wall noting masses or tenderness.			

3. Tests any stool on the gloved finger for occult blood. (For reference, go to Procedure Checklist Chapter 29: Testing Stool for Occult Blood.)			

Recommendation: Pass _____ Needs more practice _____

Student: _____ Date: _____

Instructor: _____ Date: _____

PROCEDURE CHECKLIST
Chapter 22: Assessing the Breasts and Axillae

Check (✓) Yes or No

PROCEDURE STEPS	Yes	No	COMMENTS
Before, during, and after the procedure, follows Principles-Based Checklist to Use With All Procedures, including: Identifies patient using two identifiers and according to agency policy; attends appropriately to standard precautions, hand hygiene, safety, privacy, and body mechanics.			
1. Inspects the breasts, nipples, areola, and axillae for skin condition, size, shape, symmetry, and color. Notes hair distribution in axillae.			

2. Inspects with client in these positions:
  a. Sitting or standing, arms at sides.
  b. Sitting or standing, arms raised overhead.
  c. Sitting or standing, hands pressed on the hips.
  d. Sitting or standing and leaning forward.
  e. Supine with a pillow under the shoulder of the breast being examined.			

3. Compares breasts bilaterally.			
4. Inspects nipples for discharge; if present, obtains a culture.			
5. Wearing procedure gloves as necessary, uses fingerpads of the three middle fingers to palpate the breasts using the vertical strip method, pie wedge, or concentric circles. Vertical strip method: Starts at the sternal edge and palpates the breast in parallel lines until reaching the midaxillary line. Goes up one area and down the adjacent strip (like "mowing the grass"). Pie wedge method: This method examines the breast in wedges. Moves from one wedge to the next. Concentric circles method: Starts in the outermost area of the breast at the 12 o'clock position. Moves clockwise in concentric, ever smaller, circles.			

Copyright © 2016, F. A. Davis Company, Wilkinson & Treas/Procedure Checklists for Fundamentals of Nursing, 3e

PROCEDURE STEPS	Yes	No	COMMENTS
5a. Does not remove fingers from skin surface while palpating; moves by sliding fingers along the skin.			
6. Palpates the nipples and areola. a. Notes tissue elasticity and tenderness.			
b. Squeezes nipple gently between thumb and finger to check for discharge.			
c. If open lesion or nipple discharge is present, wears procedure gloves to palpate the breasts.			
7. Palpates axillae and clavicular lymph nodes. a. Patient sitting with arms at sides, or supine.			
b. Uses fingerpads and moves fingers in circular fashion.			
c. Palpates all nodes: central, anterior pectoral, lateral brachial, posterior subscapular, epitrochlear, infraclavicular, supraclavicular.			

Recommendation: Pass _____ Needs more practice _____

Student: _____   Date: _____

Instructor: _____   Date: _____

 Copyright © 2016, F. A. Davis Company, Wilkinson & Treas/Procedure Checklists for Fundamentals of Nursing, 3e

PROCEDURE CHECKLIST
Chapter 22: Assessing the Chest and Lungs

Check (✓) Yes or No

PROCEDURE STEPS	Yes	No	COMMENTS
Before, during, and after the procedure, follows Principles-Based Checklist to Use With All Procedures, including: Identifies patient using two identifiers and according to agency policy; attends appropriately to standard precautions, hand hygiene, safety, privacy, and body mechanics.			
1. Assesses respirations by counting the respiratory rate and observing the rhythm, depth, and symmetry of chest movement.			
2. Inspects the chest for AP: lateral diameter, costal angle, spinal deformity, respiratory effort, and skin condition.			
3. Palpates trachea with fingers and thumb.			
4. Palpates the chest. 　a. Palpates for tenderness, masses, or crepitus. 　b. Places hands on chest wall: anterior, posterior, and lateral.			
5. Palpates chest excursion. 　a. Places hands at the base of the chest with fingers spread and thumbs about 2 inches (5 cm) apart (at the costal margin anteriorly and at the 8th to 10th rib posteriorly). 　b. Presses thumbs toward the spine to create a small skinfold between them. 　c. Has the client take a deep breath and feels for chest expansion.			
6. Palpates chest for tactile fremitus, using palms only.			
7. Percusses chest. 　a. Percusses over intercostal spaces rather than over bones.			
b. Uses indirect method of percussion.			
c. Percusses anterior, posterior, and lateral.			
d. Compares right side to left side.			
8. Percusses anterior chest for diaphragmatic excursion			
a. Percusses diaphragm level on full expiration; marks level.			
b. Percusses diaphragm level on full inspiration; marks level.			
c. Measures distance between the two marks.			

PROCEDURE STEPS	Yes	No	COMMENTS

9. Auscultates the chest.
   a. Using same pattern as for percussion.
   b. Using diaphragm of stethoscope.
   c. Has client take slow, deep breaths through his mouth while listening at each site through one full respiratory cycle.			

10. Auscultates for abnormal voice sounds if there is evidence of lung congestion. Correctly uses one of the following methods, following the same pattern as for auscultation:			
a. Assesses for bronchophony by having the client say "1, 2, 3" as nurse listens over the lung fields.			
b. Assesses for egophony by having client say "eee" while nurse listens over the lung fields.			
c. Assesses for whispered pectoriloquy by having client whisper "1, 2, 3" while nurse listens over the lung fields.			
11. Follows the same pattern and sequence of correctly identified landmarks when auscultating, palpating, and percussing the chest.			

Recommendation: Pass _____ Needs more practice _____

Student: _____   Date: _____

Instructor: _____   Date: _____

 Copyright © 2016, F. A. Davis Company, Wilkinson & Treas/Procedure Checklists for Fundamentals of Nursing, 3e

PROCEDURE CHECKLIST
Chapter 22: Assessing the Ears and Hearing

Check (✔) Yes or No

PROCEDURE STEPS	Yes	No	COMMENTS
Before, during, and after the procedure, follows Principles-Based Checklist to Use With All Procedures, including: Identifies patient using two identifiers and according to agency policy; attends appropriately to standard precautions, hand hygiene, safety, privacy, and body mechanics.			
1. Inspects the external ear for placement, size, shape, symmetry, drainage, lesions, and color and condition of skin.			
2. Palpates the external structures of the ear for condition of skin, lesions, and tenderness.			
3. Using otoscope, inspects tympanic membrane and bony landmarks.			
a. Uses correct size speculum.			
b. Has patient tilt head to side not being examined.			
c. Looks for foreign object in canal before inserting scope.			
d. *For Adult*: Pulls pinna up and back. *For Child*: Pulls pinna down and back.			
e. Inserts speculum slowly, no further than halfway into the ear canal.			
f. Identifies location of cone of light and bony landmarks.			
g. Uses "puff" of air to test TM mobility.			
4. Tests gross hearing. a. Stands 1 to 2 feet behind the patient. Has the patient cover one ear and then whispers some words. Repeats on the other side. Has the patient repeat the words heard.			
b. Has the patient occlude one ear. Holds a ticking watch next to the patient's unobstructed ear. Slowly moves it away until the patient says he can hear the sound.			
5. Performs Weber test (places vibrating tuning fork on top of patient's head, identifying as positive if sound not heard equally in both ears).			

PROCEDURE STEPS	Yes	No	COMMENTS
6. Performs Rinne test if Weber is positive. a. Strikes a tuning fork on the table. While it is still vibrating, places it on the patient's mastoid process. b. Measures the elapsed time in seconds that the patient hears the vibration. c. Moves the tuning fork to 1 inch (2.5 cm) in front of the ear and measures the elapsed time until the patient can no longer hear the vibration. d. Compares AC and BC times.			
7. Performs Romberg test: a. Has client stand with feet together, hands at side, with eyes opened and then with eyes closed. b. Stands near patient and notes ability to maintain balance. c. Identifies swaying as positive Romberg. (This may be deferred until the sensori-neurological exam.)			
8. Compares bilaterally throughout examination.			

Recommendation: Pass _____ Needs more practice _____

Student: _____   Date: _____

Instructor: _____   Date: _____

 Copyright © 2016, F. A. Davis Company, Wilkinson & Treas/Procedure Checklists for Fundamentals of Nursing, 3e

PROCEDURE CHECKLIST
Chapter 22: Assessing the Eyes

Check (✓) Yes or No

PROCEDURE STEPS	Yes	No	COMMENTS
Before, during, and after the procedure, follows Principles-Based Checklist to Use With All Procedures, including: Identifies patient using two identifiers and according to agency policy; attends appropriately to standard precautions, hand hygiene, safety, privacy, and body mechanics.			
1. Assesses distance vision using a Snellen chart.			
a. Chooses correct chart for age and literacy.			
b. Allows client to wear corrective lenses for test.			
c. Has patient stand 20 feet from chart and cover one eye at a time.			
d. Tests eyes singly and then together.			
e. Records findings correctly.			
2. Tests near vision by measuring the ability to read newsprint at a distance of 14 inches (35 cm). Correctly identifies hyperopia or presbyopia if present.			
3. Tests color vision by using color plates or the color bars on the Snellen chart. Follows up with Ishihara cards if needed.			
4. Assesses peripheral vision by determining when an object comes into sight.			
a. Seats client 2 to 3 feet (60 to 90 cm) from nurse.			
b. Has client cover one eye and gaze straight ahead.			
c. Begins well outside normal peripheral vision and brings object to the center of the visual fields.			
d. Repeats in all four visual fields, clockwise.			
5. Assesses EOMs by examining: a. for parallel alignment. b. the corneal light reflex. c. the ability to move through the six cardinal gaze positions. d. the cover/uncover test.			
6. Inspects external structures: a. Color and alignment of eyes.			
b. Eyelids: Notes any lesions, edema, or lid lag.			
c. Symmetry and distribution of eyelashes.			
d. Lacrimal ducts and glands, checks for edema, and drainage.			

PROCEDURE STEPS	Yes	No	COMMENTS
e. Notes color, moisture, and contour of conjunctiva.			
f. Inspects both palpebral and bulbar conjunctiva.			
g. Sclera: Notes color and presence of lesions.			
h. Inspects cornea and lens with penlight; notes color and lesions.			
i. If indicated, tests the corneal reflex with a cotton wisp or puff of air.			
j. Notes color, size, shape, and symmetry of iris and pupils.			
k. Checks pupil reaction for direct and consensual response.			
l. Assesses pupil accommodation by having the patient focus on an approaching object.			
m. Inspects anterior chamber with penlight, for color, size, shape, and symmetry.			
7. Palpates the external eye structures for tenderness and discharge; palpates globes and lacrimal glands and ducts.			
8. Assesses the internal structures via ophthalmoscopy. a. Darkens the room.			
b. Stands about 1 foot from the patient at a 15° degree lateral angle.			
c. Dials the lens wheel to zero with index finger.			
d. Holds ophthalmoscope to own brow.			
e. Has the patient look straight ahead while shining the light on one pupil to identify the red light reflex.			
f. Once the red light reflex is identified, moves in closer to within a few inches of the eye and observes the internal structures of the eye. Adjusts the lens wheel to focus as needed.			
g. Uses right eye to examine the patient's right eye, and left eye to examine the patient's left eye.			

Recommendation: Pass _____ Needs more practice _____

Student: _____   Date: _____

Instructor: _____   Date: _____

PROCEDURE CHECKLIST
Chapter 22: Assessing the Female Genitourinary System

Check (✔) Yes or No

PROCEDURE STEPS	Yes	No	COMMENTS
Before, during, and after the procedure, follows Principles-Based Checklist to Use With All Procedures, including: Identifies patient using two identifiers and according to agency policy; attends appropriately to standard precautions, hand hygiene, safety, privacy, and body mechanics.			
1. Instructs client to disrobe to expose the pelvic area.			
2. Positions patient in lithotomy or Sims position, providing support as needed.			
3. Inspects external genitalia.			
a. Notes distribution and condition of pubic hair.			
b. Inspects mons, pubis, and labia for color, lesions, and discharge.			
4. Wearing gloves, uses thumb and index finger to separate the labia and expose the clitoris; observes for size and position.			
5. With labia separated, observes urethral meatus and vaginal introitus for color, size, and presence of discharge or lesions. Then asks client to bear down while observing the introitus for bulging or discomfort.			
6. Palpates Bartholin's and Skene's glands.			
a. Lubricates gloved middle and index fingers of dominant hand with water soluble lubricant.			
b. Palpates Bartholin's gland by inserting fingers into the introitus and palpating the lower portion of the labia bilaterally between thumb and fingers.			
c. Palpates Skene's glands by then rotating the internal fingers upward and palpating the labia bilaterally.			
d. Milks the urethra by applying pressure with index finger on the anterior vaginal wall; cultures any discharge.			
7. Assesses vaginal and pelvic muscle tone by inserting two gloved fingers into the vagina and asking the woman to constrict her vaginal muscles, and then to bear down as if she is having a bowel movement.			

PROCEDURE STEPS	Yes	No	COMMENTS
8. Palpates lymph nodes in the groin area and the vertical chain over the inner aspect of the thigh.			

Recommendation: Pass _____ Needs more practice _____

Student: _____   Date: _____

Instructor: _____   Date: _____

Check (✓) Yes or No

PROCEDURE STEPS	Yes	No	COMMENTS
Before, during, and after the procedure, follows Principles-Based Checklist to Use With All Procedures, including: Identifies patient using two identifiers and according to agency policy; attends appropriately to standard precautions, hand hygiene, safety, privacy, and body mechanics.			
1. Assesses both scalp hair and body hair.			
2. Palpates hair texture.			
3. Assesses hair color, quantity, and distribution; condition of scalp; and presence of lesions or pediculosis.			
4. Inspects and palpates scalp; notes mobility, tenderness, and lesions.			

Recommendation: Pass _____ Needs more practice _____

Student: _____ Date: _____

Instructor: _____ Date: _____

Copyright © 2016, F. A. Davis Company, Wilkinson & Treas/Procedure Checklists for Fundamentals of Nursing, 3e

PROCEDURE CHECKLIST
Chapter 22: Assessing the Head and Face

Check (✔) Yes or No

PROCEDURE STEPS	Yes	No	COMMENTS
Before, during, and after the procedure, follows Principles-Based Checklist to Use With All Procedures, including: Identifies patient using two identifiers and according to agency policy; attends appropriately to standard precautions, hand hygiene, safety, privacy, and body mechanics.			
1. Compares side to side throughout the exam.			
2. Inspects head for size, shape, symmetry, and position.			
3. Inspects face for expression and symmetry.			
4. Palpates head for masses, tenderness, and scalp mobility.			
5. Palpates face for symmetry, tenderness, muscle tone, and TMJ function.			

Recommendation: Pass _____ Needs more practice _____

Student: _____   Date: _____

Instructor: _____   Date: _____

Copyright © 2016, F. A. Davis Company, Wilkinson & Treas/Procedure Checklists for Fundamentals of Nursing, 3e

PROCEDURE CHECKLIST
Chapter 22: Assessing the Heart and Vascular System

Check (✔) Yes or No

PROCEDURE STEPS	Yes	No	COMMENTS
Before, during, and after the procedure, follows Principles-Based Checklist to Use With All Procedures, including: Identifies patient using two identifiers and according to agency policy; attends appropriately to standard precautions, hand hygiene, safety, privacy, and body mechanics.			
1. Inspects the neck and chest. Positions patient supine.			
a. Observes carotid arteries and jugular veins for pulsations.			
2. Assesses jugular flow by compressing jugular vein below the jaw and observing for vein collapse and jugular wave.			
3. Assesses jugular filling by compressing jugular vein above the clavicle and observing for vein distention and disappearance of jugular wave.			

4. Measures jugular venous pressure (JVP).
   a. Elevates the head of the bed to a 45° angle.
   b. Identifies the highest point of visible internal jugular filling.
   c. Places a ruler vertically at the sternal angle (*where the clavicles meet*).
   d. Places another ruler horizontally at the highest point of the venous wave.
   e. Measures the distance in centimeters vertically from the chest wall.			

5. Places patient supine with tangential lighting to inspect precordium for pulsations.			
6. Palpates the carotid arteries, if indicated.			
a. Palpates each side separately and gently.			
b. Avoids massaging the artery.			
c. Notes rate, rhythm, amplitude, and symmetry of pulse.			
d. Notes contour, symmetry, and elasticity of the arteries; notes any thrills.			
7. Palpates the precordium for pulsations, lifts, heaves, and thrills.			
a. Has patient sit up and lean forward; if unable to sit up, turns patient to the left side.			

PROCEDURE STEPS	Yes	No	COMMENTS
b. Palpates: apex, left lateral sternal border, epigastric area, base left, and base right.			
c. Works from patient's right side to auscultate, if possible.			
8. Auscultates the carotids: uses bell of stethoscope, has patient hold his breath while listening.			
9. Auscultates jugular veins: uses bell of stethoscope, has patient hold his breath while listening.			
10. Auscultates the precordium: a. Identifies S_1, S_2, S_3, and S_4 sounds. b. Listens for murmurs. c. Listens with both bell and diaphragm at all four locations.			
d. Listens at: base right (aortic valve), base left (pulmonic valve), apex (mitral valve), and left lateral sternal border (tricuspid valve).			
11. If murmur is heard, identifies variables affecting (e.g., location, quality, pitch, intensity, timing, duration, configuration, radiation, and respiratory variation) and compares with previous findings. Refers to primary care provider if murmur is a new finding.			
12. Inspects the periphery for color, temperature, and edema.			
13. Palpates the peripheral pulses: radial, brachial, femoral, popliteal, dorsalis pedis, and posterior tibial.			
a. Uses distal pads of second and third fingers to firmly palpate pulses.			
b. Palpates firmly but does not occlude artery.			
c. Assesses pulses for rate, rhythm, equality, amplitude, and elasticity.			
d. Describes pulse amplitude on a scale of 0 to 4: 　0 = absent, not palpable 　1 = diminished, barely palpable 　2 = normal, expected 　3 = full, increased 　4 = bounding			

PROCEDURE STEPS	Yes	No	COMMENTS
14. Inspects the venous system. If a client has varicosities, assesses for valve competence with the manual compression test.			

Recommendation: Pass _____ Needs more practice _____

Student: _____ Date: _____

Instructor: _____ Date: _____

PROCEDURE CHECKLIST
Chapter 22: Assessing the Male Genitourinary System

Check (✔) Yes or No

PROCEDURE STEPS	Yes	No	COMMENTS
Before, during, and after the procedure, follows Principles-Based Checklist to Use With All Procedures, including: Identifies patient using two identifiers and according to agency policy; attends appropriately to standard precautions, hand hygiene, safety, privacy, and body mechanics.			
1. Instructs client to empty his bladder and undress to expose the groin area.			
2. Positions patient standing and sits at eye level to the genitalia; or positions patient supine with legs slightly apart.			
3. Inspects external genitalia.			
a. Notes distribution and condition of pubic hair.			
b. Inspects penis, noting condition of skin, presence or absence of foreskin, position of urethral meatus, and any lesions or discharge.			
c. Observes the scrotum for: skin condition, size, position, and symmetry.			
d. Inspects inguinal areas for swelling or bulges.			
4. Palpates penis.			
a. Uses thumb and fingers of gloved hand.			
b. Notes consistency, tenderness, masses, or nodules.			
c. Retracts foreskin if present.			
5. Palpates scrotum, testes, and epididymis.			
a. Uses thumb and fingers of gloved hand. Notes size, shape, consistency, mobility, masses, nodules, or tenderness.			
b. Transilluminates any lumps, nodules, or edematous areas by shining a pen light over the area in a darkened room.			

6. Palpates for inguinal hernias with a gloved hand.
   a. Has the patient hold his penis to one side.
   b. Places index finger in the client's scrotal sac above the testicle and invaginates the skin.
   c. Follows the spermatic cord until reaching a slitlike opening (Hesselbach's triangle).
   d. Asks the client to cough or bear down while feeling for bulges.			

PROCEDURE STEPS	Yes	No	COMMENTS
7. Palpates for femoral hernias with a gloved hand by palpating below the femoral artery while having the client cough or bear down.			
8. Palpates the lymph nodes with a gloved hand in the groin area and the vertical chain over the inner aspect of the thigh.			

Recommendation: Pass _____ Needs more practice _____

Student: _____ Date: _____

Instructor: _____ Date: _____

PROCEDURE CHECKLIST
Chapter 22: Assessing the Mouth and Oropharynx

Check (✔) Yes or No

PROCEDURE STEPS	Yes	No	COMMENTS
Before, during, and after the procedure, follows Principles-Based Checklist to Use With All Procedures, including: Identifies patient using two identifiers and according to agency policy; attends appropriately to standard precautions, hand hygiene, safety, privacy, and body mechanics.			
1. Inspects mouth externally. Notes the placement, color, and condition of lips. Asks client to purse the lips.			
2. Dons procedure gloves. Notes color and condition of oral mucosa and gums:			
a. Inspects lower lip inside and outside.			
b. Uses tongue depressor and penlight to inspect buccal mucosa, and Stensen's ducts.			
c. Palpates inside each cheek.			
d. Inspects gums for color, bleeding, edema, retraction, and lesions.			
e. Palpates gums for firmness.			
f. Palpates any lesions for size, mobility, and tenderness.			
3. Inspects teeth for color, condition, and occlusion.			
4. If client wears dentures, asks her to remove them; inspects for cracked or worn areas. Assesses for fit.			
5. Inspects tongue and floor of the mouth.			
a. Asks client to stick out his tongue. Examines upper surface for color, texture, position, and mobility.			
b. Has client place tip of tongue on roof of his mouth; uses penlight to inspect underside of tongue, frenulum, floor of mouth, submaxillary glands, and Wharton's ducts.			
c. Using tongue blade or gloved finger, moves tongue aside and examines lateral aspects of tongue and floor of mouth.			
d. Palpates tongue and floor or mouth, stabilizing the tongue by grasping with a gauze pad.			
6. Inspects the oropharynx (hard/soft palate, tonsils, and uvula); notes color, shape, texture, and condition.			
a. Has the client tilt his head back and open his mouth as widely as possible. Depresses the tongue with a tongue blade and shines a penlight on the areas to be inspected.			

PROCEDURE STEPS	Yes	No	COMMENTS
b. To inspect the uvula, asks the client to say "ah" and watches the uvula as the soft palate rises.			
c. Inspects the oropharynx by depressing one side of the tongue at a time, about halfway back on the tongue.			
d. Notes the size and color of the tonsils; notes any discharge.			
e. Inspects for cleft palate.			
7. Tests the gag reflex by touching the back of the soft palate with a tongue blade.			
8. Asks the client to repeat the following words: light, tight, dynamite. (May defer this test to the sensorineurological portion of the exam.)			

Recommendation: Pass _____ Needs more practice _____

Student: _____   Date: _____

Instructor: _____   Date: _____

    Copyright © 2016, F. A. Davis Company, Wilkinson & Treas/Procedure Checklists for Fundamentals of Nursing, 3e

PROCEDURE CHECKLIST
Chapter 22: Assessing the Musculoskeletal System

Check (✓) Yes or No

PROCEDURE STEPS	Yes	No	COMMENTS
Before, during, and after the procedure, follows Principles-Based Checklist to Use With All Procedures, including: Identifies patient using two identifiers and according to agency policy; attends appropriately to standard precautions, hand hygiene, safety, privacy, and body mechanics.			
1. Compares bilaterally during assessment.			
2. Inspects posture, body alignment, and symmetry from the front, back, and side.			

3. Assesses spinal curvature with client:
  a. Standing erect.
  b. Bending forward at waist, arms hanging free at sides.			

4. Observes position of the knees with client standing erect with feet together.			

5. Examines gait by observing client walking; notes:
  a. Base of support (distance between the feet).
  b. Stride length (distance between each step.
  c. Phases of the gait.			

6. If gait is steady, proceeds to Step 7. If unsteady, assesses balance through:
  a. Tandem walking.
  b. Heel and toe walking.
  c. Deep knee bends.
  d. Hopping.
  e. Romberg test (feet together, eyes open; then eyes closed).			

7. Assesses coordination:
  a. Assesses with client seated.
  b. Tests finger-thumb opposition.
  c. Tests rapid alternating movements by having client alternate supination and pronation of the hands.
  d. Tests rhythmic toe-tapping, one side at a time.
  e. Has client run heel of one foot down the shin of the other leg; repeats on opposite side.			

8. Tests the accuracy of movements by having the client touch his finger to his nose with his eyes open, then with eyes closed.			

PROCEDURE STEPS		Yes	No	COMMENTS
9. Measures arm length from acromion process to the tip of the middle finger.				
10. Measures apparent leg length from umbilicus to the medial malleolus.				
11. Measures true leg length from the anterior superior iliac crest, crossing over the knee to the medial malleolus.				
12. Measures circumference of forearms, upper arms, thighs, and calves.				
13. Inspects symmetry and shape of muscles and joints.				
14. Notes surgical scars indicating joint surgeries.				
15. Tests active ROM by asking client to move each of the following joints: temporomandibular, neck, thoracic and lumbar spine; shoulder, upper arm and elbow; wrist, hands, and fingers; hip, knee, ankles, and feet.				
16. Checks for the following joint movements:				
a. Temporo-mandibular	Able to flex, extend, move side-to-side, protrude, and retract the jaw.			
b. Neck	Flexes, extends, hyperextends, bends laterally, and rotates side-to-side.			
c. Thoracic and lumbar spine	Able to bend at the waist, stand upright, hyperextend (bend backward), bend laterally, and rotate side-to-side.			
d. Shoulder	Able to move the arm forward and backward, abduct, adduct, and rotate internally and externally.			
e. Upper arm and elbow	Able to bend, extend, supinate, and pronate the elbow.			
f. Wrist	Flexes, extends, hyperextends, and moves side-to-side.			
g. Hands and fingers	Able to spread the fingers (abduct), bring them together (adduct), make a fist (flex), extend the hand (extend), bend fingers back (hyperextend), and bring thumb to index finger (palmar adduction).			
h. Hip	Able to extend the leg straight, flex the knee to the chest, abduct and adduct the leg, rotate the hip internally and externally, and hyperextend the leg.			
i. Knee	Able to flex and extend the knee.			

PROCEDURE STEPS		Yes	No	COMMENTS
j. Ankles and feet	Able to dorsiflex, plantar flex, evert, invert, abduct, and adduct the feet and plantar flexion of foot, dorsiflexion of foot.			
17. Assesses muscle strength by having the client perform ROM against resistance: hand grip, biceps, triceps, legs, ankles.				
18. Rates muscle strength correctly using the following rating scale:				

18. Rates muscle strength correctly using the following rating scale:

Rating	Criteria	Classification
5	Active motion against full resistance	Normal
4	Active motion against some resistance	Slight weakness
3	Active motion against gravity	Weakness
2	Passive ROM	Poor ROM
1	Slight flicker of contraction	Severe weakness
0	No muscular contraction	Paralysis

Recommendation: Pass _____ Needs more practice _____

Student: _____   Date: _____

Instructor: _____   Date: _____

Copyright © 2016, F. A. Davis Company, Wilkinson & Treas/Procedure Checklists for Fundamentals of Nursing, 3e

PROCEDURE CHECKLIST
Chapter 22: Assessing the Nails

Check (✔) Yes or No

PROCEDURE STEPS	Yes	No	COMMENTS
Before, during, and after the procedure, follows Principles-Based Checklist to Use With All Procedures, including: Identifies patient using two identifiers and according to agency policy; attends appropriately to standard precautions, hand hygiene, safety, privacy, and body mechanics.			
1. Compares bilaterally throughout exam.			
2. Inspects nails for color, condition, texture, and shape.			
3. Palpates the texture of the nails.			
4. Correctly assesses capillary refill by pressing on the nails and releasing.			
5. States normal finding for capillary refill (less than 2 to 3 seconds).			
6. Examines nails on hands and feet, both; or states he will defer examination of the toenails until the assessment of peripheral circulation.			

Recommendation: Pass _____ Needs more practice _____

Student: _____   Date: _____

Instructor: _____   Date: _____

Copyright © 2016, F. A. Davis Company, Wilkinson & Treas/Procedure Checklists for Fundamentals of Nursing, 3e

PROCEDURE CHECKLIST
Chapter 22: Assessing the Neck

Check (✔) Yes or No

PROCEDURE STEPS	Yes	No	COMMENTS
Before, during, and after the procedure, follows Principles-Based Checklist to Use With All Procedures, including: Identifies patient using two identifiers and according to agency policy; attends appropriately to standard precautions, hand hygiene, safety, privacy, and body mechanics.			
1. Inspects the neck in both neutral and hyperextended position, and while patient swallows water.			
2. Notes symmetry, range of motion (ROM), and condition of skin.			
3. Palpates the cervical lymph nodes. a. Uses light palpation with one or two fingerpads, in a circular movement.			
b. Palpates all nodes in this order: pre-auricular, posterior auricular, tonsillar, submandibular, submental, occipital, superficial cervical, deep cervical, posterior cervical, and supraclavicular.			
c. Notes the size, shape, symmetry, consistency, mobility, tenderness, and temperature of any palpable nodes.			

4. Palpates the thyroid, using correct technique.
To use the posterior approach:
    a. Stands behind the client and asks him to flex his neck slightly forward and to the left.
    b. Positions thumbs on the nape of the client's neck.
    c. Using the fingers of the left hand, locates the cricoid cartilage. Pushes the trachea slightly to the left with the right hand while palpating just below the cricoid and between the trachea and sternocleidomastoid muscle. Asks client to swallow (gives small sips of water if necessary) and feels for the thyroid gland as it rises up.
    d. Reverses and repeats the same steps to palpate the right thyroid lobe (uses fingers of left hand to displace the trachea to the right while using the fingers of the right hand to palpate the thyroid to the right of the trachea).			

PROCEDURE STEPS	Yes	No	COMMENTS
To use the anterior approach: a. Stands in front of the client and asks him to flex his neck slightly forward and in the direction the nurse intends to palpate. b. Places hands on the neck and applies gentle pressure to one side of the trachea while palpating the opposite side of the neck for the thyroid as the client swallows. c. Reverses and repeats the same steps on the opposite side.			
5. If thyroid is enlarged, or there is a mass, follows up with auscultation of the gland.			

Recommendation: Pass _____ Needs more practice _____

Student: _____ Date: _____

Instructor: _____ Date: _____

PROCEDURE CHECKLIST
Chapter 22: Assessing the Nose and Sinuses

Check (✓) Yes or No

PROCEDURE STEPS	Yes	No	COMMENTS
Before, during, and after the procedure, follows Principles-Based Checklist to Use With All Procedures, including: Identifies patient using two identifiers and according to agency policy; attends appropriately to standard precautions, hand hygiene, safety, privacy, and body mechanics.			
1. Compares right and left sides throughout examination.			
2. Positions client sitting, if possible.			
a. Inspects the external nose, noting the position, shape, and size; discharge and flaring.			

3. Checks for patency of the nasal passages.
   a. Asks the client to close his mouth, hold one naris closed, and breathe through the other naris.
   b. Repeats with opposite naris.			

4. Inspects the internal structures. a. Holds speculum in right hand to inspect left nostril; in left hand to inspect right nostril.			
b. Tilts the client's head back to facilitate speculum insertion and visualization.			
c. Braces index finger against the client's nose while inserting the speculum.			
d. Inserts the speculum about 1 cm into the naris; opens as much as possible.			
e. Uses the other hand to position client's head and hold penlight.			
f. Observes the nasal mucosa for color, edema, lesions, and discharge.			
g. Inspects the septum for position and intactness.			
h. *Infants and children*—Does not use a speculum to examine internal structures. Pushes the tip of the nose upward with thumb and directs a penlight into the nares.			
5. Transilluminates the frontal and maxillary sinuses. a. Darkens the room.			
b. *Frontal sinuses*: Shines a penlight or the otoscope with speculum below eyebrow on each side.			

PROCEDURE STEPS	Yes	No	COMMENTS
c. *Maxillary sinuses*: Places the light source below the eyes and above the cheeks. Looks for a glow of red light at the roof of the mouth through the client's open mouth.			
6. Palpates the external structures.			
7. Palpates the frontal and maxillary sinuses.			

Recommendation: Pass _____ Needs more practice _____

Student: _____   Date: _____

Instructor: _____   Date: _____

PROCEDURE CHECKLIST
Chapter 22: Assessing the Sensory-Neurological System

Check (✓) Yes or No

PROCEDURE STEPS	Yes	No	COMMENTS
Before, during, and after the procedure, follows Principles-Based Checklist to Use With All Procedures, including: Identifies patient using two identifiers and according to agency policy; attends appropriately to standard precautions, hand hygiene, safety, privacy, and body mechanics.			
1. Assesses behavior, noting facial expression, posture, affect, and grooming.			
2. Determines level of arousal using as needed and in this order: verbal stimuli, tactile stimuli, painful stimuli.			
3. Correctly describes altered levels of arousal using the Glasgow Coma Scale or Full Outline of UnResponsiveness (FOUR).			
4. Determines level of orientation.			
a. Checks orientation to time.			
b. Checks orientation to place.			
c. Checks orientation to person.			
5. Assesses immediate, recent, and remote memory. a. Immediate memory (asks client to repeat a series of numbers, beginning with a series of three). Then repeats test, asking client to repeat numbers in reverse order.			
b. Recent memory (names thee items and asks client to recall them later in the exam; or asks "How did you get to the hospital?" and so forth).			
c. Remote memory (asks birth date, for example).			
6. Assesses mathematical and calculative skills, beginning with simplest problem and progressing to more difficult.			
a. Considers the person's language, education, and culture in deciding whether this test is appropriate for him.			
b. Uses the following tests, as appropriate: 1) Has the client solve a simple mathematical problem, such as 3 + 3. 2) If client is able to solve that problem, presents a more complex example, such as: If you have $3.00 and you buy an item for $2.00, how much money will you have left? 3) To assess both calculation skills and attention span, asks the client to count backward from 100.			

PROCEDURE STEPS	Yes	No	COMMENTS
4) A more difficult test is to have the client perform *serial threes* or *serial sevens*. Asks him to begin at 100 and keep subtracting 3 (or 7).			
7. Assesses general knowledge by asking the client how many days in the week or months in the year.			
8. Evaluates thought processes throughout the exam. Assesses attention span, logic of speech, ability to stay focused, and appropriateness of responses.			
9. Assesses abstract thinking, for example, by asking the client to interpret a proverb, such as "A penny saved is a penny earned."			
10. Assesses judgment by asking the client to respond to a hypothetical situation, such as, "If you were walking down the street and saw smoke and flame coming from a house, what would you do?"			
11. Assesses communication ability.			
a. During the exam, notes the rate, flow, choice of vocabulary, and enunciation in client's speech.			
b. Tests spontaneous speech: Shows client a picture and has him describe it.			
c. Tests motor speech by having the client say "do, re, mi, fa, so, la, ti, do."			
d. Tests automatic speech by having the client recite the days of the week.			
e. Tests sound recognition by having the client identify a familiar sound, such as clapping hands.			
f. Tests auditory-verbal comprehension by asking the client to follow simple directions (e.g., point to your nose, rub your left elbow).			
g. Tests visual recognition by pointing to objects and asking the client to identify them.			
h. Tests visual-verbal comprehension by having the client read a sentence and explain its meaning.			
i. Tests writing by having the client write his name and address.			
j. Tests ability to copy figures by having the client copy a circle, x, square, triangle and star.			
12. CN I–checks patency of nostrils, checks one nostril at a time for client's ability to identify the smell of common substances.			
13. CN II–tests visual acuity and visual fields; performs fundoscopic exam.			

 Copyright © 2016, F. A. Davis Company, Wilkinson & Treas/Procedure Checklists for Fundamentals of Nursing, 3e

PROCEDURE STEPS	Yes	No	COMMENTS

14. CN III, IV, and VI–
   a. Tests EOMs by having the client move the eyes through the six cardinal fields of gaze with the head held steady.
   b. Tests pupillary reaction to light and accommodation.			

15. CN V, motor function– has client move his jaw from side to side, clenching his jaw, and biting down on a tongue blade.			
16. CN V, sensory function–has the client close his eyes and identify when nurse is touching his face at the forehead, cheeks, and chin bilaterally—first with the finger and then with a toothpick.			
17. Tests corneal reflex, if indicated, by touching the cornea with a wisp of cotton or puffing air from a syringe over the cornea.			
18. CN VII, motor function–has the client make faces, such as a smile, frown, or whistle.			
19. CN VII, taste–tests taste on the anterior portion of the tongue by placing sweet (sugar), salty (salt), or sour (lemon) substance on tip of tongue.			

20. CN VIII–Uses:
   a. Watch-tick test for hearing.
   b. Weber and Rinne tests for air and bone conduction.
   c. Romberg test for balance (if not already done).			

21. CN IX and X–observes ability to talk, swallow, and cough.			
22. CN IX and X, motor function–asks client to say "ah" while depressing tongue with a tongue blade and observing the soft palate and uvula to rise.			
23. CN IX and X, sensory function–touches back of pharynx with tongue blade to induce a gag reflex.			
24. CN IX and X, taste (sweet, salty, sour)–tests on posterior portion of tongue.			

25. CN XI (if not assessed with musculoskeletal exam):
   a. Places hands on client's shoulders and has client shrug his shoulders against resistance.
   b. Has client turn his head from side to side against resistance.			

26. CN XII–has the client:
   a. Say "d, l, n, t."
   b. Protrude the tongue and move it from side to side.			

PROCEDURE STEPS	Yes	No	COMMENTS
27. When testing superficial sensations: a. Begins with the most peripheral part of the limb.			
b. If client does not perceive the touch, determines boundaries by testing at about every inch (2.5 cm); sketches the area of sensory loss.			
c. Waits 2 seconds before moving to a new site.			
d. Tests first with wisp of cotton, then tests for pain with toothpick or sterile needle (first the dull, then the sharp end).			
e. Alternates dull and sharp ends when moving from spot to spot.			
f. Tests temperature sensation if pain perception is abnormal.			
28. Tests deep vibratory sensation by placing a vibrating tuning fork on a metatarsal joint and distal interphalangeal joint and having the patient identify when the vibration is felt and when it stops.			
29. Tests deep kinesthetic sensation (position sense) by holding the client's finger or toe on the sides and moving it up or down. Instructs client to keep his eyes closed and identify the direction of the movement.			
30. Performs all discriminatory sensation tests: stereognosis, graphesthesia, two-point discrimination, point localization, and sensory extinction.			
31. Uses correct procedure to test discriminatory sensation tests: a. Assesses stereognosis by placing a familiar object (e.g., a coin or a button) in the palm of the client's hand and having him identify it.			
b. Assesses graphesthesia by drawing a number or letter in the palm of patient's hand and having the patient identify what was drawn.			
c. Tests two-point discrimination with toothpicks. Has the patient close his eyes. Touches him on the finger with two separate toothpicks simultaneously. Gradually moves the points together and has the patient say "one" or "two" each time the toothpicks are moved. Documents distance and location at which he can no longer feel two separate points.			

PROCEDURE STEPS	Yes	No	COMMENTS
d. Tests point localization by having the patient close his eyes while the nurse touches him. Have him point to the area touched. Repeat on both sides and upper and lower extremities.			
e. Tests sensory extinction by simultaneously touching the patient on both sides (e.g., on both hands, both knees, both arms). Has the patient identify where he was touched.			
32. Tests each of the following deep tendon reflexes: biceps, triceps, brachioradialis, patellar, and Achilles.			
33. Uses correct procedure to test each reflex: a. Biceps reflex (spinal cord level C–5 and C–6). Rests the patient's elbow in nondominant hand, with thumb over the biceps tendon. Strikes the percussion hammer to own thumb.			
b. Triceps reflex (spinal cord level C–7 and C–8). Abducts patient's arm at the shoulder and flexes it at the elbow. Supports the upper arm with nondominant hand, letting the forearm hang loosely. Strikes the triceps tendon about 1–2 inches (2.5 to 5 cm) above the olecranon process.			
c. Brachioradialis reflex (spinal cord level C–3 and C–6). Rests patient's arm on patient's leg. Strikes with the percussion hammer 1–2 inches (2.5 to 5 cm) above the bony prominence of the wrist on the thumb side.			
d. Patellar reflex (spinal cord level L–2, L–3, and L–4). Has patient sit with legs dangling. Strikes the tendon directly below the patella.			
e. Achilles reflex (spinal cord level S–1, S–2). Has the patient lie supine or sit with the legs dangling. Holds the patient's foot slightly dorsiflexed and strikes the Achilles tendon about 2 inches (5 cm) above the heel with the percussion hammer.			
34. Uses the following scale to grade reflexes: 0 No response detected +1 Diminished response +2 Response normal +3 Response somewhat stronger than normal +4 Response hyperactive with clonus			

PROCEDURE STEPS	Yes	No	COMMENTS
35. Tests plantar superficial reflex with thumbnail or pointed object. Strokes sole of foot in an arc from the lateral heel to medially across the ball of the foot.			
36. Performs mental status screening. Tests:			
a. Orientation to time, place, and person			
b. Communication, vocabulary			
c. General knowledge			
d. Word comprehension			
e. Reading comprehension			
f. Abstract reasoning			
g. Thought processes			
h. Memory			
i. Auditory comprehension, sound recognition			
j. Mathematical and calculation skills			

<u>Recommendation</u>: Pass _____ Needs more practice _____

Student: _____ Date: _____

Instructor: _____ Date: _____

 Copyright © 2016, F. A. Davis Company, Wilkinson & Treas/Procedure Checklists for Fundamentals of Nursing, 3e

PROCEDURE CHECKLIST
Chapter 22: Assessing the Skin

Check (✓) Yes or No

PROCEDURE STEPS	Yes	No	COMMENTS
Before, during, and after the procedure, follows Principles-Based Checklist to Use With All Procedures, including: Identifies patient using two identifiers and according to agency policy; attends appropriately to standard precautions, hand hygiene, safety, privacy, and body mechanics.			
1. Uses inspection, palpation, and olfaction.			
2. Assesses both exposed and unexposed areas.			
3. Compares side to side throughout exam.			
4. Inspects skin color.			
5. Notes unusual odors.			
6. Palpates skin temperature with dorsal aspect of hand or fingers.			
7. Palpates skin texture, moisture, and hydration.			
8. Inspects for edema. Notes location, degree, and type if present.			
9. Considers culture/ethnicity, gender, and developmental stage of client in interpreting data.			
10. Inspects and palpates lesions.			
11. For identified lesions, describes size, shape, color, distribution, texture, surface relationship, exudates, tenderness, or pain.			
12. Uses ABCDE method to evaluate lesions that may need referral due to potential malignancy.			

Recommendation: Pass _____ Needs more practice _____

Student: _____   Date: _____

Instructor: _____   Date: _____

Copyright © 2016, F. A. Davis Company, Wilkinson & Treas/Procedure Checklists for Fundamentals of Nursing, 3e

PROCEDURECHECKLIST
Chapter 22: Brief Bedside Assessment

Check (✓) Yes or No

PROCEDURE STEPS	Yes	No	COMMENTS
Before, during, and after the procedure, follows Principles-Based Checklist to Use With All Procedures, including: Identifies patient using two identifiers and according to agency policy; attends appropriately to standard precautions, hand hygiene, safety, privacy, and body mechanics.			
1. Greets patient; asks patient's name and checks wristband.			
2. Explains what she/he is going to do.			
3. Observes environment (e.g., IV lines, oxygen, urinary catheter).			
4. Observes patient's general appearance and signs of distress.			
5. Measures temperature, pulse, respirations, blood pressure, and pulse oximetry.			
6. Assesses all body systems using a systematic approach (e.g., head-to-toe).			
7. With each system, observes mobility, ROM, balance, and coordination.			
8. During the exam, when talking with the patient, observes thought processes and level of consciousness.			
9. Assesses the integument (hair, nails, and skin).			
a. When examining each area of the body: notes skin color, rashes, and lesions.			
—palpates for temperature, turgor, and texture.			
—inspects hair and nails in the area.			
—assesses wounds (appearance, size, drainage, dressings, drains).			
b. Inspects and palpates hair and scalp.			
10. Assesses the head and neck.			
a. External ears, hearing			
b. Eyes: Observes pupil reaction, cardinal fields of gaze, vision, color of conjunctiva			
c. Lips: Observes color, mucous membranes			
d. Tongue and oropharynx (observes hydration, color, lesions)			

PROCEDURE STEPS	Yes	No	COMMENTS

e. Carotid, if necessary
     —Palpates lightly, one side at a time.
     —Auscultates for bruits.			

11. Examines the back with patient in sitting position:			
a. Inspects skin.			
b. Auscultates breath sounds, side to side and apex to base.			
c. Notes cough, secretions, number of pillows used for sleeping, and elevation of head of bed.			
d. Checks oxygen order, SaO_2, ability to use incentive spirometer.			

12. With patient sitting and leaning forward a bit, auscultates heart sounds.
   a. Notes rate, rhythm, S_1, S_2, and extra sounds.
   b. Inquires about cardiovascular problems.			

13. Assesses the anterior chest. a. Asks about any respiratory or cardiovascular problem.			
b. Palpates skin turgor, temperature, and PMI.			
c. Auscultates breath sounds.			
14. Inspects abdomen with patient supine:			
a. Inspects for size, shape, symmetry, and condition of skin.			
b. Observes abdominal movements: respirations, pulsations, and peristalsis.			
c. Auscultates bowel sounds in all four quadrants.			
d. Auscultates aorta for bruits.			
e. Palpates all four quadrants for: tenderness, guarding, and masses.			
f. Inspects for rebound.			
g. Determines time of last bowel movement, and pattern of BMs.			
15. Assesses urinary status.			
a. Reviews voiding pattern (patient or chart), including frequency and dysuria.			
b. Observes catheter tubing for patency and kinks.			
c. Observes color of urine.			
d. Monitors I & O if indicated.			
e. Palpates for bladder distention.			
16. Assesses upper extremities, with patient sitting if possible.			

PROCEDURE STEPS	Yes	No	COMMENTS
a. Inspects the condition of the skin and nails.			
b. Palpates skin temperature.			
c. Palpates bilateral brachial and radial pulses.			
d. Checks capillary refill.			
e. Checks ROM. Notes any stiffness or limited range of motion of the hands and arms.			
f. Tests muscle strength by having the patient grip the nurse's hands or two fingers.			
g. Notes whether the patient has any casts, traction, splints, or slings.			
h. Observes for edema.			
17. Assesses lower extremities.			
a. Observes ROM and ability to ambulate or move about in bed.			
b. Inspects the condition of the skin and nails.			
c. Palpates skin temperature and pedal pulses.			
d. Checks capillary refill.			
e. Tests for leg strength by asking the patient to raise the leg against counterpressure (preferably with the patient sitting).			
f. Checks sensation through light touch, proceeding to pain as needed.			
g. Observes for problems such as paralysis.			
h. Observes for edema.			
18. Asks the patient to stand, and inspects for:			
a. Gross spinal deformities.			
b. Balance and coordination of movements.			
c. Range of motion and gait.			
19. With the patient seated in bed, legs extended, checks for:			
a. Babinski reflex.			
b. Homans' sign.			

Recommendation: Pass _____ Needs more practice _____

Student: _____   Date: _____

Instructor: _____   Date: _____

PROCEDURE CHECKLIST
Chapter 22: Performing the General Survey

Check (✓) Yes or No

PROCEDURE STEPS	Yes	No	COMMENTS
Before, during, and after the procedure, follows Principles-Based Checklist to Use With All Procedures, including: Identifies patient using two identifiers and according to agency policy; attends appropriately to standard precautions, hand hygiene, safety, privacy, and body mechanics.			
1. Observes for signs of distress and fatigue; alters approach or provides rest periods if patient is distressed.			
2. Observes apparent age, gender, and race.			
3. Notes facial characteristics, symmetry of features, expression, and condition and color of skin.			
4. Notes body type and posture.			
5. Greets patient with handshake to assess muscle strength (if culturally appropriate).			
6. Observes gait and any abnormal movements (or ability to move about in bed).			
7. Listens to speech pattern, pace, quality, tone, vocabulary, and sentence structure.			
8. Obtains interpreter if there is a language barrier.			
9. Assesses general mental state and affect.			
10. Observes dress, grooming, and hygiene.			
11. Measures vital signs.			
12. Measures height and weight. a. *Adults:* Calculates BMI from height and weight measurement.			
b. *Infants and children <2 years:* Height—positions supine with knees extended; also measures head circumference.			
c. *Infants:* Weighs without clothing. d. *Older children:* Weighs in underwear.			
13. For children, plots height and weight on growth chart and evaluates trends.			

Recommendation: Pass _____ Needs more practice _____

Student: _____ Date: _____

Instructor: _____ Date: _____

Check (✓) Yes or No

PROCEDURE STEPS	Yes	No	COMMENTS
Before, during, and after the procedure, follows Principles-Based Checklist to Use With All Procedures, including: Identifies the patient according to agency policy using two identifiers; attends appropriately to standard precautions, hand hygiene, safety, privacy, and body mechanics.			
1. Determines correct glove size.			
2. Assesses glove package for intactness and expiration date.			
3. Creates a clean space for opening the package.			
4. Opens the outer wrapper and places the glove package on a clean, dry surface.			
5. Opens the inner package so that glove cuffs are nearest to the nurse.			
6. Fully opens the package flaps so they do not fold back over and contaminate the gloves.			
7. Takes care to not touch anything else on the sterile field, with the nondominant hand grasping the inner surface of the glove for the dominant hand and lifting up and away from the table.			
8. Slides the dominant hand into the glove, keeping the hand and fingers above the waist and away from the body.			
9. Slides gloved fingers under the cuff of the glove for the nondominant hand.			
10. Lifts the glove up and away from the table and away from the body.			
11. Slides the nondominant hand into the glove, avoiding contact with the gloved hand.			
12. Adjusts both gloves to fit the fingers and so that there is no excess at the fingertips.			
13. Keeps hands between shoulder and waist level.			
(**Note:** To remove gloves, follows the procedure for removing PPE.)			

Recommendation: Pass _____ Needs more practice _____

Student: _____   Date: _____

Instructor: _____   Date: _____

Copyright © 2016, F. A. Davis Company, Wilkinson & Treas/Procedure Checklists for Fundamentals of Nursing, 3e

PROCEDURE CHECKLIST
Chapter 23: Donning Personal Protective Equipment (PPE)

Check (✓) Yes or No

PROCEDURE STEPS	Yes	No	COMMENTS
Before, during, and after the procedure, follows Principles-Based Checklist to Use With All Procedures, including: Identifies the patient according to agency policy using two identifiers; attends appropriately to standard precautions, hand hygiene, safety, privacy, and body mechanics.			
1. Assesses the need for personal protective equipment. *Gloves*: When the nurse may be exposed to potentially infectious secretions or materials. *Gowns*: When the nurse's uniform may become exposed to potentially infectious secretions. *Face mask*: When splashing may occur and potentially contaminate the nurse's mouth or nose. *Face shield or eye goggles*: When splashing may occur and potentially contaminate the nurse's eyes. *N-95 respirator*: When caring for patients infected with airborne microorganism. *Hair cover*: When there is potential for splashes or sprays of body fluids. *Shoe covers*: When there is potential for contaminating shoes with body fluids.			
2. Gathers appropriate PPE.			
3. Dons gown first. a. Picks up the gown by the shoulders; allows to fall open without touching any contaminated surface.			
b. Slips arms into the sleeves; fastens ties at the neck.			
c. If the gown does not completely cover clothing, wears two gowns. Places the first gown on with the opening in the front and then places the second gown over the first with the opening in the back.			
4. Dons a face mask or N-95 respirator. Identifies the top edge of the mask by locating the thin metal strip that goes over the bridge of the nose. a. Picks up the mask with the top ties or ear loops.			
b. Places the metal strip over the bridge of the nose and presses it so it conforms to the bridge of the nose.			
c. Ties upper ties or slips loops around the ears.			

Copyright © 2016, F. A. Davis Company, Wilkinson & Treas/Procedure Checklists for Fundamentals of Nursing, 3e

PROCEDURE STEPS	Yes	No	COMMENTS
d. Places the lower edge of the mask below the chin and ties lower ties.			
5. Dons the face shield by placing the shield over the eyes, adjusting the metal strip over the bridge of nose, and tucking the lower edge below the chin. Secures straps behind head.			
6. If using safety glasses or goggles, dons them by setting them over the top edge of the face mask.			
7. Dons hair cover (as indicated).			
8. Dons shoe covers (as indicated).			
9. Dons gloves. Selects the appropriate size.			
10. If wearing a gown, makes sure that the glove cuff extends over the cuff of the gown.			
11. If there is not complete coverage, tapes the glove cuff to the gown.			

Recommendation: Pass _____ Needs more practice _____

Student: _____   Date: _____

Instructor: _____   Date: _____

PROCEDURE CHECKLIST
Chapter 23: Donning Sterile Gown and Gloves (Closed Method)

Check (✔) Yes or No

PROCEDURE STEPS	Yes	No	COMMENTS
Before, during, and after the procedure, follows Principles-Based Checklist to Use With All Procedures, including: Identifies the patient according to agency policy; attends appropriately to standard precautions, hand hygiene, safety, privacy, and body mechanics.			
1. Grasps the gown at the neckline; allows it to fall open while stepping back from the table.			
2. Does not allow the gown to touch any nonsterile surface.			
3. Slides both arms into the sleeves without extending hands through the cuffs.			
4. Keeps the sleeves of the gown above waist level.			
5. Asks a coworker to pull up the gown shoulders and tie neck tie (coworker touches only inside of the gown).			
6. Dons sterile gloves, closed method: a. *Glove the dominant hand*: Opens the sterile glove wrapper, keeping fingers inside the sleeve of the gown.			
b. With the nondominant hand, keeping hands inside gown sleeves, grasps cuff of the glove for the nondominant hand.			
c. Turns dominant hand palm up.			
d. Places the glove on the gown cuff of the dominant forearm, thumb side down with the glove opening pointed toward the fingers, thumb of glove over the thumb-side of the dominant hand.			
e. Keeping the dominant hand inside the sleeve, grasps the inside glove cuff through the gown, being careful to keep fingers inside the gown.			
f. With the nondominant hand encased in the gown sleeve, grasps the upper side of the glove cuff and stretches it over the cuff of the gown.			
g. Pulls sleeve of gown up to assist cuff over the wrist and moves fingers into the glove.			
h. *Glove the nondominant hand:* Places the fingers of the gloved hand under the cuff of the second glove.			

PROCEDURE STEPS	Yes	No	COMMENTS
i. Places the second glove on the forearm of the nondominant hand, thumb side down with glove opening pointing toward the fingers.			
j. Anchors the inside glove cuff, through the gown, with the nondominant hand. With the dominant hand, pulls the glove cuff over the gown cuff.			
k. Adjusts the fingers in both gloves.			
7. Grasps the waist tie on the gown and hands the tie to the circulating nurse or coworker who is wearing a hair cover and mask. Coworker grabs the tie with sterile forceps. Makes a three-quarter turn and receives the tie from the coworker.			
8. Secures the waist tie.			

Recommendation: Pass _____ Needs more practice _____

Student: _____   Date: _____

Instructor: _____   Date: _____

Check (✔) Yes or No

PROCEDURE STEPS	Yes	No	COMMENTS
Before, during, and after the procedure, follows Principles-Based Checklist to Use With All Procedures, including: Identifies the patient according to agency policy using two identifiers; attends appropriately to standard precautions, hand hygiene, safety, privacy, and body mechanics.			
Using Soap and Water:			
1. Pushes up the sleeves; removes jewelry and watch.			
2. Adjusts water temperature to warm.			
3. Wets hands and wrists under running water, keeping hands lower than wrists and forearms.			
4. Avoids splashing water onto clothing.			
5. Avoids touching inside of the sink.			
6. Applies 3–5 mL liquid or foam soap.			
7. Rubs soap over all surfaces of hands.			
8. Rubs hands vigorously together for at least 15 seconds.			
9. Lathers all surfaces of the hands and fingers.			
10. Cleans under fingernails, if nails are dirty.			
11. Rinses thoroughly, keeping hands lower than forearms.			
12. Dries hands thoroughly: moves from fingers up forearms; blots with paper towel.			
13. Turns off faucet with paper towel. Does not handle the towel with the other hand.			
14. Applies recommended hand moisturizer.			
Using Alcohol-Based Handrubs:			
1. If hands are soiled, washes them with soap and water.			
2. Removes jewelry, bares arms, and so on, as with the soap-and-water procedure.			
3. Applies a sufficient quantity of antiseptic solution to cover the hands and wrists.			
4. Vigorously rubs solution on all surfaces of fingers and hands.			
5. Continues rubbing until hands are completely dry, or as recommended by the manufacturer or agency policy.			

Copyright © 2016, F. A. Davis Company, Wilkinson & Treas/Procedure Checklists for Fundamentals of Nursing, 3e

PROCEDURE STEPS	Yes	No	COMMENTS

Recommendation: Pass _____ Needs more practice _____

Student: _____   Date: _____

Instructor: _____   Date: _____

84   Copyright © 2016, F. A. Davis Company, Wilkinson & Treas/Procedure Checklists for Fundamentals of Nursing, 3e

PROCEDURE CHECKLIST
Chapter 23: Preparing and Maintaining a Sterile Fields

Check (✓) Yes or No

PROCEDURE STEPS	Yes	No	COMMENTS
Before, during, and after the procedure, follows Principles-Based Checklist to Use With All Procedures, including: Identifies patient according to agency policy using two identifiers; attends appropriately to standard precautions, hand hygiene, safety, privacy, and body mechanics.			
1. Assesses the sterility of all packages and equipment.			
2. Arranges the environment, as needed.			
3. Positions patient before setting up a sterile field (for bedside procedures).			
Preparing a Sterile Field with Commercial Package:			
4. Places the sterile package on a clean, dry surface.			
5. Opens the flaps in this order to create a sterile field: a. Opens the flap farthest from own body.			
b. Opens side flaps.			
c. Opens flap nearest body.			
6. Treats as unsterile the area 1 inch from all edges of the wrapper, and any area hanging over the edge of the table.			
Preparing a Sterile Field with Fabric or Paper-Wrapped Package:			
7. Checks and removes the chemical indicator strip.			
8. Removes the outer wrapper and places the inner package on a clean, dry surface.			
9. Opens the inner wrapper following the same technique described in Steps 4 and 5 above.			
Preparing a Sterile Drape:			
10. Places the package on a clean, dry surface.			
11. Holds the edge of the package flap down toward the table and grasps the top edge of the package and peels back.			
12. Picks up the sterile drape by the corner and allows it to fall open without touching unsterile surfaces.			
13. Places drape on a clean, dry surface, touching only the edge of the drape.			
14. Does not fan the drape.			

PROCEDURE STEPS	Yes	No	COMMENTS
Adding Supplies to a Sterile Field:			
15. Holds the package in the dominant hand and uses the nondominant hand to peel back the wrapper in which the item is wrapped, creating a sterile barrier field with the inside of the wrapper.			
16. Holding the contents through the wrapper, several inches above the field, allows the supplies to drop onto the field inside the 1-inch border of the sterile field.			
17. Does not let arms pass over the sterile field; does not touch supplies with nonsterile hands.			
18. Disposes of the wrapper and continues opening any needed supplies for the procedure.			
Adding Sterile Solutions to a Sterile Field:			
19. If the sterile field is fabric or otherwise at risk for strikethrough, uses a sterile bowl or receptacle. It may be added to the field by unwrapping as described in the preceding section.			
20. Places a sterile bowl near the edge of the sterile field.			
21. Checks that the sterile solution is correct and not expired.			
22. Removes the cap from the solution bottle by lifting directly up.			
23. If the cap will be reused, sets it upside down on a clean area.			
24. Holds the bottle of solution 4–6 inches above the bowl to pour needed amount into the bowl.			
25. Before donning sterile gloves to perform the procedure, checks to see that all supplies have been added to the field.			
Note:			
26. Does not leave a sterile field unattended or outside the field of vision.			

Recommendation: Pass _____ Needs more practice _____

Student: _____   Date: _____

Instructor: _____   Date: _____

PROCEDURE CHECKLIST
Chapter 23: Removing Personal Protective Equipment (PPE)

Check (✓) Yes or No

PROCEDURE STEPS	Yes	No	COMMENTS
Before, during, and after the procedure, follows Principles-Based Checklist to Use With All Procedures, including: Identifies the patient according to agency policy using two identifiers; attends appropriately to standard precautions, hand hygiene, safety, privacy, and body mechanics.			
Removes PPE in the following order:			
1. If wearing a gown that is tied in front, unties waist ties. Otherwise, begins at Step 2.			
2. Removes gloves. (If gown is tied in back, removes gloves first.) a. Removes one glove by grasping the cuff of the glove and pulling down so the glove turns inside out. Holds the glove removed in the remaining gloved hand.			
b. Slips the fingers of the ungloved hand inside the cuff of the other glove; pulls glove off inside out, turning it over to enclose the first glove. Does not touch self with the contaminated surface of either glove.			
c. Holds the contaminated gloves away from the body.			
d. Disposes of gloves in a designated waste receptacle.			
3. Removes gown. a. Releases neck and waist ties of gown, allowing the gown to fall forward.			
b. Slips hands inside the gown neck and peels down off arms so that the inside of the gown faces outward.			
c. Reaches inside to pull off the cuff and remove the arm from the sleeve, one arm at a time. Does not touch the front of the gown.			
d. Holding the gown away from body, folds inside-out and discards. Does not contaminate clothing with the dirty gown.			
(**Note:** If wearing two gowns, the second gown is removed now.)			
4. Removes goggles before the mask. Grasps by earpieces.			
5. Removes the mask or face shield by untying lower ties first; unties upper ties next; disposes in designated waste receptacle. Does not touch the front of the mask.			

PROCEDURE STEPS	Yes	No	COMMENTS
6. Removes hair covering. Slips fingers under the edge of the hair cover; does not touch the outside of it. Disposes of hair cover properly.			
7. Removes shoe covers, if wearing them.			
8. Washes hands before leaving the room.			
9. Closes the door on leaving.			

Recommendation: Pass _____ Needs more practice _____

Student: _____   Date: _____

Instructor: _____   Date: _____

PROCEDURE CHECKLIST
Chapter 23: Surgical Hand Washing (Brushless System)

Check (✓) Yes or No

PROCEDURE STEPS	Yes	No	COMMENTS
Before, during, and after the procedure, follows Principles-Based Checklist to Use With All Procedures, including: Identifies the patient according to agency policy using two identifiers; attends appropriately to standard precautions, hand hygiene, safety, privacy, and body mechanics.			
1. Follows agency policy for length of scrub and type of cleansing agent used (scrub typically takes 2–5 minutes).			
2. Before starting the scrub, gathers supplies and sets up sterile gown, gloves, and towel for use after the scrub.			
3. Follows agency policy regarding fingernail polish, artificial nails, and nail length.			
4. Removes rings, watch, and bracelets.			
5. Dons surgical shoe covers, cap, and face mask before the scrub.			
Pre-wash:			
6. Performs a pre-wash before the surgical scrub.			
7. Removes debris from under the nails, using a nail pick under running water.			
Surgical Scrub Using Antimicrobial Soap:			
8. Turns on water using knee or foot controls.			
9. Adjusts water temperature to warm.			
10. Wets hands and forearms from elbows to fingertips.			
11. Keeps hands above elbows and away from body.			
12. Dispenses a palmful of antibacterial solution into the dominant hand.			
13. Inserts fingertips of the nondominant hand into cleansing solution, using a twisting motion to apply to fingertips and nails.			
14. Rubs hands together to distribute cleansing solution over them.			
15. Does not touch the inside of the sink.			
16. Vigorously rubs all surfaces of the nondominant hand and fingers as follows, adding water as needed.			

PROCEDURE STEPS	Yes	No	COMMENTS
17. Rubs hands together, palm to palm.			
18. Using the dominant palm, cleans the back of the nondominant hand. Then rubs the nondominant palm over the dominant hand.			
19. Then rubs the palms together with the fingers interlaced.			
20. Rubs the back of the fingers on the closed dominant hand and rubs them back and forth across the nondominant palm, with the fingers interlaced. Repeats with the other hand.			
21. Using a rotational movement, clasps the dominant thumb with the nondominant hand. Repeats on the other thumb.			
22. Holds the fingers together on the dominant hand and moves them back and forth and in a circular pattern against the other palm, and vice versa.			
23. Rinses and dispenses soap into the hands each time when cleansing a new area.			
24. Cleanses the remaining two-thirds of the nondominant arm to 2 inches above the elbow, covering every aspect of the arm. Rinses the arm.			
25. Repeats the wrist-to-elbow scrub on the dominant arm. Rinses thoroughly, each arm independently.			
26. Repeats all scrub steps (12–22) on both hands and arms stopping before the elbow. Usually this requires a 3-minute scrub.			
27. Arms flexed, hands higher than elbows, grasps sterile towel and backs away from sterile field.			
28. Leans forward slightly and allows towel to fall open, being careful not to let it touch the uniform.			
29. Uses one end of the towel to dry one hand and arm; uses the opposite end to dry the other hand and arm.			
30. Makes certain skin is thoroughly dry before donning sterile gloves.			

Recommendation: Pass _____ Needs more practice _____

Student: _____   Date: _____

Instructor: _____   Date: _____

PROCEDURE CHECKLIST
Chapter 23: Surgical Hand Washing (Traditional Method)

Check (✔) Yes or No

PROCEDURE STEPS	Yes	No	COMMENTS
Before, during, and after the procedure, follows Principles-Based Checklist to Use With All Procedures, including: Identifies the patient according to agency policy using two identifiers; attends appropriately to standard precautions, hand hygiene, safety, privacy, and body mechanics.			
1. Follows agency policy for length of scrub and type of cleansing agent used (scrub typically takes 2–6 minutes).			
2. Follows agency policy regarding fingernail polish, artificial nails, and nail length.			
3. Removes rings, watch, and bracelets.			
4. Dons surgical shoe covers, cap, and face mask before the scrub.			
5. Determines that sterile gloves, gown, and towel are set up for use after the scrub.			
Pre-wash:			
6. Performs a pre-wash before the surgical scrub.			
7. Removes debris from under the nails, using a nail file under running water.			
Surgical Scrub Using Antimicrobial Soap:			
8. Turns on water using knee or foot controls.			
9. Adjusts water temperature to warm.			
10. Wets hands and forearms from elbows to fingertips.			
11. Keeps hands above elbows and away from the body.			
12. Wets sponge and applies a liberal amount of soap to sponge and hands (unless sponge is pre-soaped).			
13. Lathers well to 2 inches above the elbow.			
14. Does not touch the inside of the sink.			
15. Does not splash surgical attire.			
16. Using a circular motion, scrubs all the surfaces of one hand and arm, keeping hands higher than elbows.			
17. Scrubs at least 10 strokes on each nail, all sides of fingers, and each side of the hand. Uses at least 10 strokes each for the lower, middle, and upper areas of the forearm.			
18. Rinses brush and reapplies antimicrobial soap. Repeats scrub on the other hand and arm.			

PROCEDURE STEPS	Yes	No	COMMENTS
19. Rinses hands and arms, keeping fingertips higher than elbows.			
20. Repeats Steps 12–19 if directed to do so by the soap manufacturer or agency policy.			
21. Arms flexed, hands higher than elbows, grasps sterile towel and backs away from sterile field.			
22. Leans forward slightly and allows the towel to fall open, being careful not to let it touch the uniform.			
23. Uses one end of the towel to dry one hand and arm; uses the opposite end to dry the other hand and arm.			
24. Makes certain skin is thoroughly dry before donning sterile gloves.			
(Alternatively: Uses antibacterial gel, per agency policy.)			
Surgical Scrub Using Alcohol-Based Surgical Scrub Product:			
25. Uses the indicated amount.			
26. Rubs on all surfaces of hands, nails, and arms to 2 inches above the elbow.			
27. Allows the hand-rub to dry completely before donning sterile gloves.			

Recommendation: Pass _____ Needs more practice _____

Student: _____   Date: _____

Instructor: _____   Date: _____

PROCEDURE CHECKLIST
Chapter 24: Using a Bed Monitoring Device

Check (✓) Yes or No

PROCEDURE STEPS	Yes	No	COMMENTS
Before, during, and after the procedure, follows Principles-Based Checklist to Use With All Procedures, including: Identifies the patient according to agency policy using two identifiers; attends appropriately to standard precautions, hand hygiene, safety, privacy, and body mechanics.			
1. Selects the correct type of alarm for patient.			
2. Explains to patient/family what the device is for.			
3. Mounts the control unit to the bed; alternatively, places sensor pads in the appropriate position (e.g., under patient's buttocks, on horizontal part of the leg).			
4. Connects the control unit to the sensor pad.			
5. Connects the control unit to the nurse call system, if possible.			
6. Disconnects or turns off alarm before assisting patient out of bed or chair.			
7. Reactivates the alarm after assisting patient back to bed or chair.			
8. Before leaving the room, ensures that patient has easy access to the call light.			
9. Institutes increased observation/monitoring.			

Recommendation: Pass _____ Needs more practice _____

Student: _____   Date: _____

Instructor: _____   Date: _____

Copyright © 2016, F. A. Davis Company, Wilkinson & Treas/Procedure Checklists for Fundamentals of Nursing, 3e

PROCEDURE CHECKLIST
Chapter 24: Using Restraints

Check (✓) Yes or No

PROCEDURE STEPS	Yes	No	COMMENTS
Before, during, and after the procedure, follows Principles-Based Checklist to Use With All Procedures, including: Identifies the patient according to agency policy using two identifiers; attends appropriately to standard precautions, hand hygiene, safety, privacy, and body mechanics.			
1. Follows agency policy, state laws, and Medicare standards for using restraints, as applicable.			
2. Tries alternative interventions first (e.g., bed alarm, patient sitter).			
3. Uses least invasive method of restraint that is likely to be effective.			
4. Determines that one of the following applies. Patient: a. Is a danger to self or others.			
b. Must be immobilized temporarily to perform a procedure.			
5. Obtains a medical prescription before restraining, except in an emergency.			
6. Notifies the family.			
7. Obtains written consent.			
Applying Restraints:			
8. Obtains the properly sized restraint.			
9. Pads bony prominences before applying the restraint.			
10. Secures straps in a way that allows for quick release.			
11. Does not tie restraints to the bed rail; ties to the bed frame or chair frame.			
12. Adjusts restraint to maintain good body alignment, comfort, and safety.			
13. Assesses that restraints are snug enough to prevent them from slipping off, but not tight enough to impair blood circulation or skin integrity (e.g., should be able to slide two fingers under a wrist or ankle restraint).			
Caring for a Patient in Restraints:			
14. Checks restraints every 30 minutes.			
15. Checks that a prescriber reassesses and reorders restraints every 24 hours.			

PROCEDURE STEPS	Yes	No	COMMENTS
16. Releases restraints and assesses every 2 hours (more often for behavioral restraints); provides skin care, range of motion, ambulation, and toileting.			
17. At least every 2 hours, assesses circulation, skin integrity, and need for continuing restraint.			

Recommendation: Pass _____ Needs more practice _____

Student: _____ Date: _____

Instructor: _____ Date: _____

PROCEDURE CHECKLIST
Chapter 25: Bathing: Providing a Complete Bed Bath Using a
Prepackaged Bathing Product

Check (✔) Yes or No

PROCEDURE STEPS	Yes	No	COMMENTS
Before, during, and after the procedure, follows Principles-Based Checklist to Use With All Procedures, including: Identifies the patient according to agency policy using two identifiers; attends appropriately to standard precautions, hand hygiene, safety, privacy, body mechanics, and documentation.			
1. Closes privacy curtains and drapes patient to provide privacy and prevent chilling.			
2. Assists with elimination, as needed.			
3. Asks patient and family if they wish family members to help with the bath.			
4. Peels open the label on the commercial bath without completely removing it.			
5. Takes from warmer unit, or heats in microwave for no longer than 1 minute. Temperature should be approximately 105°F (41°C).			
6. Adjusts the bed to working height, lowers siderail on the working side.			
7. Positions patient supine close to edge of bed on the working side.			
8. Removes soiled linens without exposing patient or contaminating own clothing.			
9. Removes patient's gown without exposing patient; exposes just the part of the body being bathed.			
10. If patient has an IV, removes the gown first from the arm without the IV; replaces gown on the affected arm first; does not disconnect the IV tubing (unless there is a two-way needleless connector present that allows for disconnecting and still maintaining a closed line); keeps IV container above level of patient's arm.			
11. Dons nonsterile gloves if exposure to body fluids is likely.			

PROCEDURE STEPS	Yes	No	COMMENTS

12. Uses one wipe for each body area; discards each wipe after use. In this order:
   Eyes, face, neck, and ears (uses pH-balanced wipes for eyes, or gauze moistened with water or normal saline, per agency policy)
   Arms
   Chest
   Abdomen
   Legs and feet
   Back and buttocks
   Rectal area
   Perineum			

13. Modifies the procedure or stops temporarily if patient becomes tired.			
14. Follows principle of "head to toe."			
15. Follows principle of "clean to dirty."			
16. Washes extremities from distal to proximal.			
17. Supports joints when bathing.			
18. Allows areas to air-dry; does not rinse.			
19. Dons clean procedure gloves to wash the rectal area; removes any fecal matter with tissues before using a wipe.			
20. Removes soiled gloves, performs hand hygiene, dons clean gloves, and uses a clean wipe to wash the perineal area.			
21. After bathing the back, provides a back rub if not contraindicated.			
22. Applies deodorant, lotion, and/or powder as desired or as needed.			
23. When finished, repositions patient.			
24. Changes bed linen as needed.			
25. Properly bags soiled linens.			

Recommendation: Pass _____ Needs more practice _____

Student: _____ Date: _____

Instructor: _____ Date: _____

 Copyright © 2016, F. A. Davis Company, Wilkinson & Treas/Procedure Checklists for Fundamentals of Nursing, 3e

PROCEDURE CHECKLIST
Chapter 25: Bathing: Using a Basin and Water

Check (✓) Yes or No

PROCEDURE STEPS	Yes	No	COMMENTS
Before, during, and after the procedure, follows Principles-Based Checklist to Use With All Procedures, including: Identifies the patient according to agency policy using two identifiers; attends appropriately to standard precautions, hand hygiene, safety, privacy, body mechanics, and documentation.			
1. Fills a disposable basin with warm, not hot, water (approximately 105°F [41°C]), according to agency policy for use of tap water. Checks water temperature with thermometer or hand.			
2. Adds rinse-free soap, if available. Prepares a CHG and water bathing solution, according to agency policy.			
3. Pulls the privacy curtain and drapes patient to provide privacy and prevent chilling.			
4. Adjusts the bed to working height and lowers the siderail on which the nurse begins the bath.			
5. Always raises the siderail when leaving the bed or moving to the other side.			
6. Changes water before cleansing the perineum or whenever the water is dirty or cool.			
7. Dons nonsterile gloves if exposure to body fluids is likely.			
8. Removes soiled linens without exposing patient or contaminating own clothing.			
9. Removes patient's gown without exposing patient; exposes just the part of the body being bathed.			
10. If patient has an IV, removes the gown first from the arm without the IV; replaces the gown on the affected arm first. (If a two-way needleless connector is present, may disconnect the tubing to remove the gown.)			
11. Folds the washcloth around the hand to make a bath mitt.			
12. Uses one washcloth for each body area.			
13. Rinses washcloth and wrings dry often enough to keep it warm and clean.			
14. Rinses well if using soap.			

PROCEDURE STEPS	Yes	No	COMMENTS
15. Bathes the patient's body in this order: Eyes, face, neck, and ears Arms Chest Abdomen Legs and feet Back and buttocks Rectal area Perineum			
16. Modifies procedure or stops temporarily if patient becomes tired.			
17. Follows principle of "head to toe."			
18. Follows principle of "clean to dirty."			
19. Washes extremities from distal to proximal.			
20. While bathing patient, keeps loose ends of the washcloth from dragging across the skin and wrings out excess water.			
21. Supports joints when bathing.			
22. Pats dry to protect the skin.			
23. Dries thoroughly between the toes.			

24. When washing the rectal area:
  a. Dons procedure gloves.
  b. Positions patient on his side or prone.
  c. Removes any fecal matter with tissues before using the washcloth.
  d. Removes gloves, performs hand hygiene, and dons clean gloves before proceeding with the rest of the procedure (i.e., backrub, perineal care)			

25. Applies deodorant, lotion, and/or powder as desired or as needed. Applies emollients.			
26. After washing the back, provides a back rub if not contraindicated.			
27. When finished, repositions and covers patient, and changes bed linen as needed.			
28. Bags soiled linens appropriately for laundering.			
29. Removes and discards gloves and performs hand hygiene.			

 Copyright © 2016, F. A. Davis Company, Wilkinson & Treas/Procedure Checklists for Fundamentals of Nursing, 3e

PROCEDURE STEPS	Yes	No	COMMENTS
30. Cleans basin with a CHG solution, wipes dry, and stores the basin upside down, or according to agency policy. Does not store bath or other supplies in the bath basin.			

Recommendation: Pass _____ Needs more practice _____

Student: _____   Date: _____

Instructor: _____   Date: _____

Copyright © 2016, F. A. Davis Company, Wilkinson & Treas/Procedure Checklists for Fundamentals of Nursing, 3e

PROCEDURE CHECKLIST
Chapter 25: Bathing: Providing a Towel Bath

Check (✓) Yes or No

PROCEDURE STEPS	Yes	No	COMMENTS
Before, during, and after the procedure, follows Principles-Based Checklist to Use With All Procedures, including: Identifies the patient according to agency policy using two identifiers; attends appropriately to standard precautions, hand hygiene, safety, privacy, body mechanics, and documentation.			
1. Places folded bath blanket, bath towel, and two or three washcloths in large plastic bag.			
2. Fills pitcher with approximately 2,000 mL of warm distilled, sterile, or filtered water; adds nonrinse soap or commercial solution to the water; and pours solution into the bag over the bath blanket, towel, and washcloths.			
3. Uses warm, not hot, water (105°F [41°C]).			
4. If not planning to change the linen, works one dry blanket under patient.			
5. Places a dry bath blanket over patient and pulls down bed linens, without exposing patient.			
6. Removes patient's gown without exposing patient.			
7. If patient has an IV, removes the gown first from the arm without the IV; replaces gown on the affected arm first. (If the IV tubing has a two-way needleless connector that maintains a closed line, it is acceptable to disconnect the tubing to remove the gown.)			
8. Replaces the dry blanket with a wet blanket: a. Squeezes out excess water so it does not drip.			
b. Pushes the dry blanket down to patient's waist and places the wet blanket on the chest; continues to unfold wet blanket in this manner, keeping the dry blanket dry.			
9. If necessary, places another dry blanket on top of the wet one.			
10. Bathes patient beginning at the feet and working toward the head.			
11. Uses the wet blanket to wash legs, abdomen, and chest.			

PROCEDURE STEPS	Yes	No	COMMENTS
12. As bathing is done, replaces the wet blanket with the dry one, folding the wet blanket as each area is bathed to allow only clean surfaces to contact new body areas.			
13. Uses one washcloth to wash patient's face, neck, and ears.			
14. Dons procedure gloves (if not already wearing them). Rolls patient to one side and uses a wet towel to wash the back and then the buttocks.			
15. Washes the rectal area; removes any fecal matter with tissues before using the washcloth.			
16. Changes procedure gloves; washes hands.			
17. Using washcloths, provides perineal care.			
18. Supports joints when bathing.			
19. Pats dry with dry towel, as needed; dries thoroughly between the toes.			
20. Applies deodorant, lotion, and/or powder as desired or as needed.			
21. Provides a back rub if not contraindicated.			
22. When finished, repositions patient, and changes bed linen as needed.			

Recommendation: Pass _____ Needs more practice _____

Student: _____   Date: _____

Instructor: _____   Date: _____

 Copyright © 2016, F. A. Davis Company, Wilkinson & Treas/Procedure Checklists for Fundamentals of Nursing, 3e

PROCEDURE CHECKLIST
Chapter 25: Brushing and Flossing the Teeth

Check (✓) Yes or No

PROCEDURE STEPS	Yes	No	COMMENTS
Before, during, and after the procedure, follows Principles-Based Checklist to Use With All Procedures, including: Identifies the patient according to agency policy, using two identifiers; attends appropriately to standard precautions, hand hygiene, safety, privacy, body mechanics, and documentation.			
1. Uses water from the faucet or uses filtered, sterile, or distilled water according to agency policy.			
2. Positions patient to prevent aspiration (sitting or side-lying), as needed.			
3. Sets up suction, if needed.			
4. For self-care, arranges supplies within patient's reach and assists only as needed.			
Nurse-Administered Brushing and Flossing:			
5. Places a towel across patient's chest.			
6. Dons procedure gloves, and other protective gear as needed.			
7. Adjusts the bed to working height and lowers the near siderail.			
8. Moistens the toothbrush and applies a small amount of toothpaste			
9. Places, holds, or has patient hold the emesis basin under his chin.			
10. Brushes teeth, holding bristles at a 45° angle: a. Uses short, circular motions.			
b. Brushes all surfaces of the teeth from gum line to crown.			
c. If patient is frail or at risk for choking, suctions secretions as needed.			
d. Gently brushes patient's tongue.			
11. Flosses teeth using floss holder or by the following technique: a. Wraps one end of the floss around the middle finger of each hand.			
b. Stretches the floss between thumbs and index fingers and moves the floss up and down against each tooth.			

PROCEDURE STEPS	Yes	No	COMMENTS
c. Flosses between and around all teeth.			
12. Assists patient in rinsing his mouth, suctioning as needed if patient is frail. Or asks patient to rinse vigorously and spit the water into the emesis basin.			
13. Offers a mild or dilute mouthwash and applies lip moisturizer if desired.			
14. Repositions patient as needed and returns the bed to the low position.			

Recommendation: Pass _____ Needs more practice _____

Student: _____   Date: _____

Instructor: _____   Date: _____

PROCEDURE CHECKLIST
Chapter 25: Caring for Artificial Eyes

Check (✓) Yes or No

PROCEDURE STEPS	Yes	No	COMMENTS
Before, during, and after the procedure, follows Principles-Based Checklist to Use With All Procedures, including: Identifies the patient according to agency policy using two identifiers; attends appropriately to standard precautions, hand hygiene, safety, privacy, body mechanics, and documentation.			
1. Washes hands and dons procedure gloves.			
2. Positions patient lying down.			
3. Removes the artificial eye: a. Raises the upper lid with the nondominant hand; depresses the lower lid with the dominant hand.			
b. Applies slight pressure below the eye.			
c. Catches the prosthesis in the palm of the dominant hand.			
d. Alternatively, uses a small bulb syringe to create suction on the prosthesis; lifts straight up from the socket.			
4. Cleans the eye with saline or distilled, sterile, or filtered water, according to agency requirements; does not use solvents, disinfectants, or alcohol.			
5. If storing the eye, places in a labeled container of saline or tap water.			
6. Wipes the edge of the eye socket with a moistened cotton ball, from outer canthus toward the nose.			
7. Inspects the socket for redness, swelling, or drainage.			
8. Reinserts the eye: a. Makes sure it is wet.			
b. Holds the prosthesis with the dominant hand.			
c. With the nondominant hand, pulls down on lower lid while lifting the upper lid; guides the eye into the socket.			

Recommendation: Pass _____ Needs more practice _____

Student: _____   Date: _____

Instructor: _____   Date: _____

Copyright © 2016, F. A. Davis Company, Wilkinson & Treas/Procedure Checklists for Fundamentals of Nursing, 3e

PROCEDURE CHECKLIST
Chapter 25: Caring for Hearing Aids

Check (✓) Yes or No

PROCEDURE STEPS	Yes	No	COMMENTS
Before, during, and after the procedure, follows Principles-Based Checklist to Use With All Procedures, including: Identifies the patient according to agency policy using two identifiers; attends appropriately to standard precautions, hand hygiene, safety, privacy, body mechanics, and documentation.			
Removing, Cleaning, and Reinserting a Hearing Aid:			
1. Dons procedure gloves.			
2. Places a towel on the overbed table or other flat surface.			
3. To remove: a. Turns off the hearing aid.			
b. Rotates the earmold forward and gently pulls it out.			
c. Does not pull on the battery door or volume wheel.			
4. Cleans the external surfaces of the hearing aid with a damp cloth. Does not immerse the hearing aid in water.			
5. Uses a wax-loop and wax brush, pipe cleaner, cotton-tipped applicator, or toothpick to clean the top part of the canal portion of the hearing aid. Does not insert anything into the hearing aid itself.			
Variation: For Detachable Earmold: Disconnects the earmold, soaks in soapy water, rinses and dries well, reattaches.			
6. Checks the aid and tubing for cracks and loose connections.			
7. Cleanse the outer ear with a washcloth or cotton-tipped applicator.			
8. Inspects the ear for redness, abrasions, swelling, drainage, and so on.			
9. To reinsert the hearing aid: a. Checks that battery is functioning.			
b. Closes the battery compartment door; turns power on.			

PROCEDURE STEPS	Yes	No	COMMENTS
c. Turns the volume on high and listens for a whistling sound.			
d. Sets the control volume to "off."			
e. Handles the hearing aid by the edges, with thumb and forefinger			

f. Positions correctly:
    Postaural hearing aid: Inserts the earmold first and then places the earmold over the ear.
    In-the-canal hearing aid: Inserts with the volume control at the top, canal facing away from the hand.
    In-the-ear hearing aid: Inserts with the volume control at the bottom.			

g. Uses the nondominant hand to pull the ear up and back. Inserts the canal portion of the aid into the ear, rotating the aid back and forth until the canal portion rests flat in the ear.			
h. Turns hearing aid on and adjusts the volume, setting volume as low as possible. Checks with patient.			
Storing the Hearing Aid:			
10. Opens the battery compartment and places the hearing aid in a closed container labeled with patient's name.			
11. If the aid is to be stored for a week or more, removes the battery completely.			
12. Stores in a cool, dry place (e.g., bedside drawer) away from children and pets.			
Replacing the Battery:			
13. Uses a finger to swing battery door open. Does not force it.			
14. Peels the tab off the new battery; holds with positive (+) side up and slides into the door (not into the hearing aid itself).			
15. Gently closes the door; does not force it.			
16. Disposes of the old battery in the regular trash.			

Recommendation: Pass _____ Needs more practice _____

Student: _____   Date: _____

Instructor: _____   Date: _____

Check (✓) Yes or No

PROCEDURE STEPS	Yes	No	COMMENTS
NOTE: This checklist is designed to evaluate making an occupied bed separately from giving a bed bath. If linen change is done at the same time as the bed bath, some of these steps will vary.			
Before, during, and after the procedure, follows Principles-Based Checklist to Use With All Procedures, including: Identifies the patient according to agency policy using two identifiers; attends appropriately to standard precautions, hand hygiene, safety, privacy, body mechanics, and documentation.			
1. Prepares the environment, as needed: a. Moves furniture to allow access to the bed.			
b. Positions the linen hamper for easy access.			
2. Dons protective gloves and other gear if necessary.			
3. Positions the bed flat if possible, and raises to the appropriate working height. Lowers the siderail nearest the nurse.			
4. Disconnects the call device and removes patient's personal items from the bed.			
5. Checks that no tubes are entangled in the bed linens.			
6. Leaves the siderail down only on the side of the bed where the nurse is standing. Does not walk to the other side with the rail still down.			
7. Removes blanket and/or bedspread; if clean, folds and places on a clean area. Does not place clean linen on another patient's bed or furniture.			
8. Covers patient with a bath blanket, if available, or leaves the top sheet over patient.			
9. Positions patient: a. Slides patient to the far side of the bed; places in a side-lying position facing the siderail.			
b. Places a pillow under patient's head; if needed, places a pillow between patient and the siderail.			
10. Rolls or tightly fanfolds the soiled linens toward patient's back; tucks the roll slightly under patient.			
11. Covers any moist areas of the soiled linen with a waterproof pad.			

PROCEDURE STEPS	Yes	No	COMMENTS
12. Removes soiled gloves; performs hand hygiene; and dons clean procedure gloves.			
13. Places a clean bottom sheet and drawsheet on near side of the mattress, with the center vertical fold at the center of the bed.			
14. Fanfolds the half of the clean linen that is to be used on the far side, folding it as close to the patient as possible and tucking it under the dirty linen.			
15. Tucks the lower edges of the clean linen under the mattress. Smoothes out all wrinkles.			
16. Explains to patient that he will be rolling over a "lump."			
17. Rolls patient over dirty linen and gently pulls patient toward the nurse so patient rolls onto the clean linen, side-lying, near the edge of the bed.			
18. Raises the siderail and moves pillows to the clean side of the bed.			
19. Moves to opposite side of bed; lowers the bed rail.			
20. Pulls soiled linen away from patient from under the clean linen. Removes from the bed and places in a laundry bag or hamper without contaminating the uniform.			
21. Does not put soiled linen on the floor or other surfaces.			
22. Removes soiled gloves, performs hand hygiene, and dons clean procedure gloves.			
23. Pulls clean linens through to the unmade side of the bed, and tucks them in.			
24. Pulls linens taut, starting with the middle section.			
25. Assists patient to a supine position close to the center of the mattress.			
26. Places the top sheet and bedspread along one side of the mattress; removes the bath blanket.			
27. Tucks sheet and blanket in at the same time, then moves to the opposite side of the bed.			
28. After making both sides of the bed, at the head of the bed, folds sheet down over the bedspread.			
29. At the foot of the bed, makes a small toe pleat in the top sheet and bedspread; then tucks in the bottom of the sheet and bedspread at the same time.			
30. Miters corners neatly.			

PROCEDURE STEPS	Yes	No	COMMENTS
31. Changes pillowcases: Turns inside out; grasps the middle of the closed end of the pillowcase; reaches through the pillowcase and grasps the end of the pillow; pulls the pillow back through the pillowcase. Does not hold the pillow under an arm or the chin.			
32. Returns the bed to a low position, raises siderails, and attaches the call light within patient's reach.			
33. Positions the bedside table and overbed table within patient's reach.			

Recommendation: Pass _____ Needs more practice _____

Student: _____   Date: _____

Instructor: _____   Date: _____

PROCEDURE CHECKLIST
Chapter 25: Making an Unoccupied Bed

Check (✓) Yes or No

PROCEDURE STEPS	Yes	No	COMMENTS
Before, during, and after the procedure, follows Principles-Based Checklist to Use With All Procedures, including: Identifies the patient according to agency policy using two identifiers; attends appropriately to standard precautions, hand hygiene, safety, privacy, body mechanics, and documentation.			
1. Assists patient to the chair; provides a robe/blanket if needed.			
2. Prepares the environment: a. Positions the bed flat, raises to working height, and lowers siderails.			
b. Moves furniture as needed.			
c. Places the linen hamper for convenient access.			
3. Dons procedure gloves and protective gear if necessary.			
4. Loosens all bedding.			
5. Folds and places clean bedspread and/or blanket on clean area. Does not place clean linen on another patient's bed or furniture.			
6. Removes all sheets and pillowcases; places in a laundry bag or hamper without contaminating uniform. a. Does not shake or "fan" linens.			
b. Does not place linens on the floor.			
c. Removes and replaces linens on one side of the bed at a time, to save steps.			
d. Holds soiled linen away from uniform.			
7. Replaces clean linens. For a flat bottom sheet, allows at least 10 inches to hang over at top and sides for tuck-in.			
8. Smoothes wrinkles from the bottom sheet.			
9. If there is a draw sheet, tucks it and draws it tight.			
10. Replaces the waterproof pad if one is being used.			
11. Places the top sheet and bedspread along one side of the mattress; unfolds.			
12. Makes a small pleat in the top sheet and bedspread, at the foot of the bed (toe pleat).			

PROCEDURE STEPS	Yes	No	COMMENTS
13. Tucks the top sheet and bedspread in at the same time, using a mitered corner. Then moves to the opposite side of the bed.			
14. After making both sides of the bed, at the head of the bed, folds the sheet down over the bedspread.			
15. Fanfolds the top sheet and bedspread back to the foot of the bed.			
16. Changes pillowcases: a. Turns the pillowcase wrong side out.			
b. Grasps the middle of the closed end of the pillowcase.			
c. Reaches through the pillowcase and grasps the end of the pillow.			
d. Pulls the pillow back through the pillowcase.			
e. Does not hold the pillow under an arm or the chin.			
17. Assists patient back to bed.			
18. Places the call signal within reach; puts the bed in a low position.			
19. Places the bedside table and overbed table so they are accessible to patient.			

Recommendation: Pass _____ Needs more practice _____

Student: _____   Date: _____

Instructor: _____   Date: _____

PROCEDURE CHECKLIST
Chapter 25: Providing Beard and Mustache Care

Check (✓) Yes or No

PROCEDURE STEPS	Yes	No	COMMENTS
Before, during, and after the procedure, follows Principles-Based Checklist to Use With All Procedures, including: Identifies the patient according to agency policy using two identifiers; attends appropriately to standard precautions, hand hygiene, safety, privacy, body mechanics, and documentation.			
1. Drapes a towel around patient's shoulders.			
2. Trims the beard and mustache when dry.			
3. Trims conservatively, cutting too little rather than too much: a. If using comb and scissors, cuts the hair on the outside of the comb.			
b. If using a beard trimmer, adjusts the guide to the correct length.			
4. Trims the beard from in front of the ear to the chin on one side, then repeats on the other.			
5. Mustache: Combs straight down, then starts in the middle and trims first toward one side of the mouth, then the other. Does not trim the top of the mustache.			
6. Defines the beard line with the scissors or a beard trimmer; or shaves the neck to define the beard line.			
7. Applies gloves, if needed, before shampooing the facial hair.			
8. Shampoos facial hair as needed, following agency policy for use of water; rinses well; dries with a towel. Applies conditioner if patient desires.			
9. Combs the beard and mustache with a wide-toothed comb or brush.			

Recommendation: Pass _____ Needs more practice _____

Student: _____   Date: _____

Instructor: _____   Date: _____

Copyright © 2016, F. A. Davis Company, Wilkinson & Treas/Procedure Checklists for Fundamentals of Nursing, 3e

PROCEDURE CHECKLIST
Chapter 25: Providing Denture Care

Check (✓) Yes or No

PROCEDURE STEPS	Yes	No	COMMENTS
Before, during, and after the procedure, follows Principles-Based Checklist to Use With All Procedures, including: Identifies the patient according to agency policy using two identifiers; attends appropriately to standard precautions, hand hygiene, safety, privacy, body mechanics, and documentation.			
1. Uses water from the faucet, or uses filtered, sterile, or distilled water according to agency policy.			
2. Dons procedure gloves.			
3. Removes the upper denture before the lower denture.			
4. To remove the upper denture, with a gauze pad, grasps the denture with a thumb and forefinger and moves gently up and down. Tilts the denture slightly to one side to remove it without stretching the lips.			
5. To remove lower denture, uses thumbs to gently push up on denture at gum line to release from lower jaw. Grasps the denture with thumb and forefinger and tilts to remove from patient's mouth.			
6. Places each denture in a denture cup after removing.			
7. Places a towel or basin of water in the sink to prevent damage to dentures.			
8. Cleanses the dentures under cool running water (from the faucet or poured from a cup; see Step 1).			
9. Applies a small amount of denture paste to stiff-bristled toothbrush; brushes all surfaces of each denture; rinses thoroughly with cool water. **Alternatively**, soaks stained dentures in a commercial cleaner, following the manufacturer's instructions.			
10. Inspects dentures for rough, worn, or sharp edges before replacing.			
11. Inspects the mouth under the dentures for redness, irritation, lesions, or infection before replacing dentures.			
12. Applies denture adhesive as needed or as desired by patient.			

PROCEDURE STEPS	Yes	No	COMMENTS
13. If the patient does not wish to wear the dentures, places them in a container with a lid and covers them with distilled, sterile, or filtered water. Labels container with patient's name and identifying number. Places container in a bedside drawer, not on top of the bedside table.			
14. Replaces the upper denture before the lower denture.			
15. Moistens the upper denture, if dry; inserts at a slight tilt, and presses it up against the roof of the mouth.			
16. Moistens the bottom denture, if dry; inserts the denture, rotating it as it is placed in patient's mouth.			
17. Asks the patient whether the dentures are comfortable.			
18. Offers mouthwash.			

Recommendation: Pass _____ Needs more practice _____

Student: _____ Date: _____

Instructor: _____ Date: _____

PROCEDURE CHECKLIST
Chapter 25: Providing Foot Care

Check (✔) Yes or No

PROCEDURE STEPS	Yes	No	COMMENTS
Before, during, and after the procedure, follows Principles-Based Checklist to Use With All Procedures, including: Identifies the patient according to agency policy using two identifiers; attends appropriately to standard precautions, hand hygiene, safety, privacy, body mechanics, and documentation.			
1. Wears procedure gloves as needed.			
2. Asks the patient to sit in a chair or places in semi-Fowler's position with a pillow under the knees.			
3. Places waterproof pad or bath towel under the feet and basin.			
4. Fills a disposable basin half-full with warm distilled, sterile, or filtered water (approximately 105°–110°F [40°–43°C]), according to agency policy.			
5. Inspects feet thoroughly for skin integrity, circulation, and edema; checks between toes.			
6. Soaks each foot, one at a time, for 5–20 minutes as tolerated (contraindicated for patients with diabetes or peripheral vascular disease).			
7. Changes water between feet.			
8. Cleans feet with mild soap; cleans toenails with orange stick while foot is still in the water; pushes cuticles back with orangewood stick.			
9. Rinses (or uses rinse-free soap) and dries well (especially between the toes).			
10. Trims nails straight across with toenail clippers, unless contraindicated by patient's condition or by institutional policy.			
11. Files nails with an emery board.			
12. Lightly applies cream, lotion, or foot powder. Does not apply cream or lotion between the toes.			
13. Ensures that footwear and bedding are not irritating to patient's feet; applies protective devices, if needed. Uses a bed cradle if patient has an injury, lesions, pain, or is at high risk for impaired skin integrity.			

Recommendation: Pass _____ Needs more practice _____

Student: _____   Date: _____

Instructor: _____   Date: _____

Copyright © 2016, F. A. Davis Company, Wilkinson & Treas/Procedure Checklists for Fundamentals of Nursing, 3e

PROCEDURE CHECKLIST
Chapter 25: Providing Oral Care for an Unconscious Patient

Check (✓) Yes or No

PROCEDURE STEPS	Yes	No	COMMENTS
Before, during, and after the procedure, follows Principles-Based Checklist to Use With All Procedures, including: Identifies patient according to agency policy using two identifiers; attends appropriately to standard precautions, hand hygiene, safety, privacy, body mechanics, and documentation.			
1. Determines whether patient has dentures or partial plate; assesses the gag reflex.			
2. Positions patient in a side-lying position with head turned to the side, if possible, and with head of bed down (slightly dependent, if possible).			
3. Dons procedure gloves, eye goggles, and any other protective gear needed.			
4. Places waterproof pad and then towel under patient's cheek and chin.			
5. Sets up suction: Attaches tubing and tonsil-tip suction, checks suction.			
6. Brushes patient's teeth: a. Uses a padded tongue blade or bite-block to hold the mouth open.			
b. Places an emesis basin under patient's cheek.			
c. Moistens a toothbrush with sterile, distilled, or filtered tap water according to agency requirements, and applies a small amount of toothpaste.			
d. Brushes teeth, holding bristles at a 45° angle to the gum line.			
e. Uses short, circular motions.			
f. Gently brushes the inner and outer surfaces of the teeth, including the gum line.			
g. Brushes the biting surface of the back teeth by holding the toothbrush perpendicular to the teeth and brushing back and forth.			
h. Brushes patient's tongue.			
i. Provides denture care, if necessary.			
j. Performs oral suctioning when fluid accumulates in the mouth.			

Copyright © 2016, F. A. Davis Company, Wilkinson & Treas/Procedure Checklists for Fundamentals of Nursing, 3e

PROCEDURE STEPS	Yes	No	COMMENTS
7. Draws about 10 mL of distilled, sterile, or filtered water or mouthwash (e.g., dilute hydrogen peroxide) into a syringe; ejects it gently into the side of the mouth. Allows the fluid to drain out into the basin; or suctions as needed.			
8. Cleans the tissues in the oral cavity according to agency policy. a. Uses foam swabs or a moistened gauze square wrapped around a tongue blade.			
b. Uses a clean swab for each area of the mouth: cheeks, tongue, roof of the mouth, and so forth.			
9. Removes and disposes of the basin, dries face and mouth, applies water-soluble lip moisturizer.			
10. Removes the waterproof pad and towel.			
11. Turns off suction equipment.			
12. Discards gloves and used supplies.			
13. Repositions patient as needed.			
14. Cleans and stores reusable oral hygiene tools in clean containers, separate from other articles of personal hygiene.			

Recommendation: Pass _____ Needs more practice _____

Student: _____   Date: _____

Instructor: _____   Date: _____

PROCEDURE CHECKLIST
Chapter 25: Providing Perineal Care

Check (✓) Yes or No

PROCEDURE STEPS	Yes	No	COMMENTS
Before, during, and after the procedure, follows Principles-Based Checklist to Use With All Procedures, including: Identifies the patient according to agency policy using two identifiers; attends appropriately to standard precautions, hand hygiene, safety, privacy, body mechanics, and documentation			
1. Adjusts room temperature; assists with elimination as needed.			
2. Warms the prepackaged wipes in the microwave for no longer than 1 minute. (The temperature of the contents should be approximately 105°F [41°C]).			
3. Positions patient supine.			
4. Places waterproof pads under patient.			
5. Wears procedure gloves and other protective gear as needed.			
6. Drapes patient for privacy: a. Female patient: Drapes legs and perineum using triangular-folded sheet or bath blanket.			
b. Male patient: Drapes chest with towel; drapes upper legs with another towel; leaves bed linens over lower legs. Exposes only the perineum.			
7. Removes any fecal material with toilet paper.			
8. If prepackaged wipes are not available, moistens a washcloth with water in the basin or sprays perineum with the perineal wash bottle.			
9. For females: a. Washes the perineum from front to back.			
b. Uses a clean portion of the wipe for each stroke.			
c. Cleanses the labial folds and around the urinary catheter if one is in place.			
10. For males: a. Retracts the foreskin, if present.			
b. Cleanses the head of the penis using a circular motion.			
c. Replaces foreskin and finishes washing the shaft of the penis, using firm strokes.			

PROCEDURE STEPS	Yes	No	COMMENTS
d. Washes the scrotum, using a clean portion of the wipe with each stroke.			
e. Handles the scrotum gently to avoid discomfort.			
11. Cleanses skinfolds thoroughly and allows areas to air-dry. Does not rinse.			
12. Discards each wipe after use.			
13. If perineal care is not being done as part of the bath, also cleans the anal area by asking the patient to turn to the side and washing, rinsing, and drying the area as needed.			
14. Applies skin protectants as needed. Uses powder only if patient requests it.			
15. If patient has an indwelling catheter, provides special catheter care as prescribed by agency policy. Dons clean gloves before special catheter care.			
16. Repositions and covers patient.			
17. Removes and appropriately discards soiled gloves.			
18. Changes bed linens as needed.			

Recommendation: Pass _____ Needs more practice _____

Student: _____   Date: _____

Instructor: _____   Date: _____

PROCEDURE CHECKLIST
Chapter 25: Removing and Caring for Contact Lenses

Check (✔) Yes or No

PROCEDURE STEPS	Yes	No	COMMENTS
Before, during, and after the procedure, follows Principles-Based Checklist to Use With All Procedures, including: Identifies the patient according to agency policy using two identifiers; attends appropriately to standard precautions, hand hygiene, safety, privacy, body mechanics, and documentation.			
1. Performs hand hygiene and dons gloves.			
2. Instills one to two drops of contact lens wetting solution.			
3. Removes the lens.			
Hard or gas-permeable lens: a. Places finger on patient's lower eyelid; applies gentle pressure to move lens into position; places index finger at outer corner of eye and pulls sideways; positions other hand below the eye to catch the lens. Asks patient to blink. b. Alternatively, uses suction-cup remover or pulls top eyelid up and lower lid down and then presses lower eyelid up against bottom of the lens, tipping it slightly; then moves the eyelids together.			
Soft contact lens: a. Holds eye open with nondominant hand; places tip of index finger on the lens and slides it down off the pupil. Using thumb and index finger, pinches lens and lifts it straight up off the eye.			
b. If edges of lens stick together, moistens with wetting solution and rubs until edges separate.			
4. Cleans the lens according to instructions, using lens cleaner or sterile saline.			
5. Treats lens gently so as not to tear it.			
6. Rinses lens with lens solution or sterile saline.			
7. Places lenses in a contact lens case containing soaking solution or sterile saline.			

Recommendation: Pass _____ Needs more practice _____

Student: _____   Date: _____

Instructor: _____   Date: _____

Copyright © 2016, F. A. Davis Company, Wilkinson & Treas/Procedure Checklists for Fundamentals of Nursing, 3e

Check (✓) Yes or No

PROCEDURE STEPS	Yes	No	COMMENTS
Before, during, and after the procedure, follows Principles-Based Checklist to Use With All Procedures, including: Identifies the patient according to agency policy using two identifiers; attends appropriately to standard precautions, hand hygiene, safety, privacy, body mechanics, and documentation.			
1. With input from patient, as able, identifies hair care products preferred for the procedure.			
2. If lesions or infestation are present, dons procedure gloves at this step.			
3. If possible, elevates the head of the bed.			
4. Places a bath towel or protective pad under patient's shoulders.			
5. Works fingers through patient's hair or combs hair to remove tangles before washing. If patient has her hair in small braids, does not take out the braids to wash the hair. Handles black curly hair gently, as it is fragile.			
Shampooing the Hair for a Patient on Bedrest—Using Rinse-Free Shampoo:			
Follows Steps 1–5.			
6. Applies rinse-free shampoo to thoroughly wet the hair.			
7. Works through hair, from scalp down to ends.			
8. Combs or brushes hair to remove tangles, starting at the ends and working toward the scalp.			
9. Dries hair with a bath towel.			
10. When finished, ensures that patient's linens are dry.			
11. Washes and stores brushes and combs.			
Shampooing the Hair Using Rinse-Free Shampoo Cap:			
Follows Steps 1–5.			
12. Warms the shampoo cap using a water bath or microwave, according to package instructions.			
13. Checks the temperature before placing on patient's head.			
14. Places the cap on patient's hair and massages gently.			
15. Completes hair care according to the patient's needs (see Steps 8–11).			

PROCEDURE STEPS	Yes	No	COMMENTS
Shampooing the Hair Using Basin and Water:			
Follows Steps 1–5, in last section.			
16. Unless contraindicated, lowers the head of the bed; removes the pillow from under patient's neck, and places it under her shoulders.			
17. Brings warm, not hot, water in a container to the bedside. (Uses water recommended by agency policy.)			
18. Places a shampoo tray under patient's shoulders (or head, depending on how the tray is made). a. If using a hard plastic tray, liberally pads with towels.			
b. An inflatable shampoo tray needs minimal padding.			
c. If no tray is available, improvises with a bedpan that is never used for other than hair care; pads it liberally.			
d. Ensures that the tray will drain into the washbasin or other receptacle.			
19. Folds the top linens down to patient's waist and covers her upper body with a bath blanket.			
20. Washes patient's hair. a. Wets the hair using warm water, then applies shampoo and lathers well.			
b. Works from the scalp out and from the front to the back of the head.			
c. Gently lifts patient's head to rub the back of the head.			
21. Rinses thoroughly.			
22. If desired, applies conditioner to the hair. Rinses if needed.			
23. Removes the tray and blots hair dry with a towel. Does not use circular motions to dry the hair.			
24. Combs or brushes hair to remove tangles, starting at the ends and working toward the scalp.			
25. If desired, dries hair with a hair dryer at a medium or low temperature.			
26. When finished, ensures that patient's clothing and linens are dry.			
27. Washes the shampoo tray, brushes, and combs.			
Variation: Shampooing the Hair of African-American Clients:			
28. Follows Steps 1 through 4 above.			

 Copyright © 2016, F. A. Davis Company, Wilkinson & Treas/Procedure Checklists for Fundamentals of Nursing, 3e

PROCEDURE STEPS	Yes	No	COMMENTS
29. If the hair is in cornrows or braids, does not take out the braids to wash the hair.			
30. Handles patient's hair very gently, being careful not to pull on the hair.			
31. When shampooing, threads fingers through the hair from the scalp out to the ends. Does not massage the hair in circular motions.			
32. Rinses thoroughly and then applies a conditioner on the hair.			
33. Does not use a brush or fine-toothed comb on patient's hair. Uses a wide-toothed comb or hair pick: a. Parts the hair into four sections and, using a wide-toothed comb or hair pick, begins combing near the ends of the hair, working through each section.			
b. Uses additional moisturizer or a natural oil to help soften and ease combing.			
c. Lets hair air-dry, if possible.			

Recommendation: Pass _____ Needs more practice _____

Student: _____ Date: _____

Instructor: _____ Date: _____

PROCEDURE CHECKLIST
Chapter 25: Shaving a Patient

Check (✓) Yes or No

PROCEDURE STEPS	Yes	No	COMMENTS
Before, during, and after the procedure, follows Principles-Based Checklist to Use With All Procedures, including: Identifies the patient according to agency policy using two identifiers; attends appropriately to standard precautions, hand hygiene, safety, privacy, body mechanics, and documentation.			
1. Uses the patient's chosen shaving method (e.g., safety or electric razor).			
2. Dons procedure gloves.			
3. Uses sterile, distilled, or filtered tap water according to agency requirements.			
4. Places a warm, damp face towel on the patient's face for 1–3 minutes.			
5. Applies shaving lotion with fingers or shaving brush; lathers well for 1 2 minutes.			
6. Shaves the patient: a. Pulls skin taut with the nondominant hand.			
b. If using a safety razor, holds blade at a 45° angle.			
c. Gently pulls razor across the skin.			
d. Shaves the face and neck in the same direction as hair growth.			
e. Uses short strokes.			
f. Begins at sideburns and works down to the chin on each side; then shaves the neck; last, shaves chin and upper lip.			
7. Rinses razor frequently while shaving.			
8. When finished, rinses the patient's face with cool water and gently pats dry.			
9. Applies after-shave lotion if the patient desires.			
10. Disposes of a single-use razor in a sharps container.			
11. If using a multiuse razor, shakes it to remove excess moisture and stores in a covered container. Does not dry the razor with a towel or bang it against objects.			

Recommendation: Pass _____ Needs more practice _____

Student: _____   Date: _____

Instructor: _____   Date: _____

Copyright © 2016, F. A. Davis Company, Wilkinson & Treas/Procedure Checklists for Fundamentals of Nursing, 3e   **133**

PROCEDURE CHECKLIST
Chapter 26: Medication Guidelines:
Steps to Follow for All Medications, Regardless of Type or Route

Check (✓) Yes or No

PROCEDURE STEPS	Yes	No	COMMENTS
Before, during, and after the procedure, follows Principles-Based Checklist to Use With All Procedures, including: Identifies the patient according to agency policy using two identifiers; attends appropriately to standard precautions, hand hygiene, safety, privacy, body mechanics, and documentation.			
1. *First Check*: For the patient name, patient identifier, medication, dose, route, time, and drug allergies. Checks MAR and determines when medications are due.			
2. Verifies the prescription, which should include the patient's name, patient identifier, medication name, dose, route, time, and patient allergies.			
3. Follows agency policies for medication administration, including the time frame. Does not pre-pour medications.			
4. Performs hand hygiene.			
5. Accesses patient's medication drawer. Unlocks medication cart or logs onto the medication dispensing computer.			
6. Obtains narcotic cabinet key (or code). Signs out medication when administering a narcotic or barbiturate; includes patient's name, drug dose, and other pertinent information per agency policy. Notes drug count when removing a narcotic.			
7. Selects the prescribed medication and compares with the MAR for the first five rights (patient, drug, dose, route, time).			
8. Checks for drug allergies.			
9. Checks patient identification band.			
10. Calculates dosage accurately.			
11. Checks the expiration date of all medications.			
12. Does a *Second Check* after preparing medications; verifies the correct medication, dose, route, and time.			

PROCEDURE STEPS	Yes	No	COMMENTS
13. Locks the medication cart.			

14. Administers the medications:
   a. Takes the medication and MAR into patient's room.
   b. Identifies patient by using two forms of identification, according to agency policy.
   c. Performs *Third Check.*
   d. Performs any assessments needed.
   e. Explains role to patient; teaches about each medication.
   f. Administers medication using appropriate technique.
   g. Remains with patient until each medication is taken.
   h. Documents medication in patient's MAR.			

Recommendation: Pass _____ Needs more practice _____

Student: _____ Date: _____

Instructor: _____ Date: _____

PROCEDURE CHECKLIST
Chapter 26: Adding Medications to Intravenous Fluids

Check (✓) Yes or No

PROCEDURE STEPS	Yes	No	COMMENTS
Before, during, and after the procedure, follows Principles-Based Checklist to Use With All Procedures, including: Identifies the patient according to agency policy using two identifiers; attends appropriately to standard precautions, hand hygiene, safety, privacy, body mechanics, and documentation.			
1. Determines the compatibility of the prescribed medication(s) and IV solution.			
2. Calculates or verifies amount of medication to be instilled into the IV solution and the rate of administration.			
3. Removes any protective covers and inspects bag/bottle for leaks, tears, or cracks.			
4. Using the appropriate technique, draws up the prescribed medication. (See the checklist Preparing and Drawing Up Medication: and Mixing Medications From Two Vials, as needed.) Alternatively, inserts a VAD transfer device into the medication vial.			
5. Scrubs all surfaces of IV additive port with alcohol or chlorhexadine gluconate (CHG) alcohol combination product.			
6. Removes the cap from the syringe, inserts the needle or the needleless vial access device into the injection port, and injects the medication into the bag, maintaining aseptic technique.			
7. Mixes the IV solution and medication by gently turning the bag from end to end.			
8. Places label on bag so that it can be read when the bag is hung; includes medication name, dose, route, preparer's name. Makes sure label does not cover solution label or volume marks.			
Adding Medication to an Infusing IV:			
1. Determines compatibility of medication added to existing solution.			

PROCEDURE STEPS	Yes	No	COMMENTS
2. Notes volume remaining in existing IV amount needed for dilution of medication.			
3. Clamps the running IV line.			
4. Scrubs all surfaces of IV additive port with antimicrobial swab.			
5. Removes cap from syringe; inserts safety needle or needleless vial access device into injection port; injects medication in IV bag; maintains aseptic technique.			
6. Mixes IV solution and medication by gently turning bag from end to end. Maintains bag above the level of patient's IV insertion site; does not invert drip chamber.			
7. Places label on bag so that it can be read when bag is hung. Label does not cover solution or volume marks.			
8. Unclamps IV line, runs IV at prescribed rate.			
9. Disposes of used equipment, syringe, or needleless access device, appropriately.			

Recommendation: Pass _____ Needs more practice _____

Student: _____   Date: _____

Instructor: _____   Date: _____

 Copyright © 2016, F. A. Davis Company, Wilkinson & Treas/Procedure Checklists for Fundamentals of Nursing, 3e

PROCEDURE CHECKLIST
Chapter 26: Administering Intradermal Medications

Check (✔) Yes or No

PROCEDURE STEPS	Yes	No	COMMENTS
Before, during, and after the procedure, follows Principles-Based Checklist to Use With All Procedures, including: Identifies the patient according to agency policy using two identifiers; attends appropriately to standard precautions, hand hygiene, safety, privacy, body mechanics, and documentation.			
1. Draws up medication from vial.			
2. Selects the site for injection (usual sites are the ventral surface of the forearm and upper back; upper chest may also be used).			
3. Assists patient to a comfortable position. If using a forearm, instructs patient to extend and supinate arm on a flat surface. If using the upper back, instructs patient to a prone position or to lean forward over a table or the back of a chair.			
4. Dons clean procedure gloves.			
5. Cleanses the injection site with an alcohol prep pad, or other antiseptic swab. For alcohol, circles from the center of the site outward. For CHG products, uses a back and forth motion. Allows the site to dry before administering the injection.			
6. Holds the syringe between the thumb and index finger of the dominant hand parallel to skin; removes the needle cap.			
7. Using the nondominant hand, holds the patient's skin taut by one of the following methods:			
a.If using a forearm, may be able to place a hand under the arm and pull the skin tight with thumb and fingers.			
b.Stretching skin between thumb and index finger.			
c.Pulling the skin toward the wrist or down with one finger.			
8. While continuing to hold the skin taut with the nondominant hand, holds the syringe in the dominant hand with the bevel up and parallel to patient's skin at a 5° to 15° angle.			
9. Inserts the needle slowly and advances approximately 3 mm (⅛ in.) so that the entire bevel is covered. The bevel should be visible just under the skin.			

PROCEDURE STEPS	Yes	No	COMMENTS
10. Does not aspirate. Holds syringe stable with nondominant hand.			
11. Releases the taut skin and slowly injects the solution. A pale wheal, about 6–10 mm (¼ in.) in diameter, should appear over needle bevel.			
12. Removes the needle from the skin, engages the safety needle device, and disposes in a biohazard puncture-proof container. If there is no safety device, places the uncapped syringe and needle directly in a biohazard puncture-proof container.			
13. Gently blots any blood with a dry gauze pad. Does not rub or cover with an adhesive bandage.			
14. With a pen, draws a 1-in. circle around the bleb/wheal.			

Recommendation: Pass _____ Needs more practice _____

Student: _____   Date: _____

Instructor: _____   Date: _____

PROCEDURE CHECKLIST
Chapter 26: Administering Intramuscular Injections

Check (✓) Yes or No

PROCEDURE STEPS	Yes	No	COMMENTS
Before, during, and after the procedure, follows Principles-Based Checklist to Use With All Procedures, including: Identifies the patient according to agency policy using two identifiers; attends appropriately to standard precautions, hand hygiene, safety, privacy, body mechanics, and documentation.			
1. Selects appropriate syringe and needle, considering volume and type. a. Usual syringe size is 1–3 mL.			
b. Usual needle is 21–25-gauge, 1–3-inch length for adults.			
2. Draws up medication or obtains the prescribed unit dose and verify medication with the order.			
3. Dons clean procedure gloves.			
4. Positions patient so the injection site is accessible and patient is able to relax the appropriate muscles. Assures adequate lighting. *Deltoid site:* Positions patient with arm relaxed at side or resting on a firm surface and completely exposes the upper arm. *Ventrogluteal site:* Positions patient on the side with upper hip and knee slightly flexed. *Vastus lateralis:* Positions patient supine or sitting, if the patient prefers. *Rectus femoris:* Positions patient supine. Uses only if all other sites are inaccessible and no other route is feasible.			
5. Uses appropriate landmarks. Identifies the correct injection site. If patient receives more than one injection, rotates sites.			
6. Vigorously scrubs the injection site with an antiseptic prep pad. Places prep pad on patient's skin outside injection site, with a corner pointing to the site. Allows the site to dry before administering the injection.			
7. Removes the needle cap.			

Copyright © 2016, F. A. Davis Company, Wilkinson & Treas/Procedure Checklists for Fundamentals of Nursing, 3e

PROCEDURE STEPS	Yes	No	COMMENTS
Traditional Intramuscular Method:			
8. Using the nondominant hand, holds the skin taut by spreading the skin between the thumb and index finger.			
9. Tells patient he will feel a prick as the needle is inserted. Holds the syringe between thumb and fingers of the dominant hand like a pencil or dart, and inserts the needle at a 90° angle to the skin surface. Inserts the needle fully.			
10. Stabilizes the syringe with the nondominant hand.			
11. Aspirates by pulling back on the plunger, and waits for 5–10 seconds. If blood returns, removes needle, discards, prepares medication again. If no blood returns, continue with Step 11.			
12. Using thumb or index finger of dominant hand, presses plunger slowly and injects medication (5–10 seconds/mL).			
13. Removes needle smoothly along the line of insertion.			
14. Engages safety needle device, and disposes in a biohazard container. If there is no safety device, places uncapped syringe and needle directly in a biohazard puncture-proof container.			
15. Gently blots site with gauze pad, applies light pressure and adhesive bandage as needed.			
16. Watches for adverse reactions at the site; reassesses in 10 to 30 minutes.			
Z-Track Administration:			
1–7. Follows steps of Traditional Intramuscular Method.			

8.   Z-track variation: Uses one of the following large muscles.
    a.   Ventrogluteal site: Positions patient on the side with the upper hip and knee slightly flexed.
    b. Vastus lateralis: Positions patient supine or sitting.			

9. With the side of the nondominant hand, displaces the skin away from the injection site, about 2.5–3.5 cm (1–1.5 in.).			
10. Holding the syringe between the thumb and fingers of the dominant hand like a pencil or dart, inserts needle at a 90° angle to the skin surface. Inserts needle fully.			

PROCEDURE STEPS	Yes	No	COMMENTS
11. Stabilizes syringe with thumb and forefinger of the nondominant hand. Does not release the skin to stabilize the syringe.			
12. Aspirates by pulling back slightly on plunger for 5–10 seconds. If blood returns, removes needle, discards, prepares medication again.			
13. Using thumb or index finger of the dominant hand, presses the plunger slowly to inject medication (5–10 seconds/mL).			
14. Waits 10 seconds, then withdraws needle smoothly along the line of insertion; immediately releases the skin.			
15. Engages the safety needle device and disposes in a biohazard container. If there is no safety device, places uncapped syringe and needle directly in a biohazard puncture-proof container.			
16. Holds cotton ball with light pressure over injection site. Does not massage injection site. Applies an adhesive bandage if necessary.			

Recommendation: Pass _____ Needs more practice _____

Student: _____   Date: _____

Instructor: _____   Date: _____

Copyright © 2016, F. A. Davis Company, Wilkinson & Treas/Procedure Checklists for Fundamentals of Nursing, 3e

PROCEDURE CHECKLIST
Chapter 26: Administering IV Push Through
Primary IV Line

Check (✓) Yes or No

PROCEDURE STEPS	Yes	No	COMMENTS
Before, during, and after the procedure, follows Principles-Based Checklist to Use With All Procedures, including: Identifies the patient according to agency policy using two identifiers; attends appropriately to standard precautions, hand hygiene, safety, privacy, body mechanics, and documentation.			
1. Determines rate of administration for medication, and compatibility with solution infusing.			
2. Prepares medication from vial, ampule, or prescribed unit dose. Verifies medication with the order.			
3. Dilutes medication if needed. Temporarily pauses infusion pump to administer medication.			
4. Dons procedure gloves.			
5. Thoroughly scrubs all surfaces of the injection port closest to the patient with the alcohol prep pad or CHG-alcohol combination product.			
6. Inserts medication syringe into injection port. If a needleless system is not available, uses syringe with a safety needle.			
7. Pinches or clamps the IV tubing between the IV bag and the port.			
8. Gently aspirates by pulling back on the plunger, and checks for blood return. (Some connectors neither require nor allow for aspiration; follow agency policy.)			
9. If blood returns on aspiration, administers a small amount of the medication while observing for reactions to the medication.			
10. Administers another increment of the medication (may pinch the tubing while injecting the medication, and release it when not injecting; this is optional).			
11. Repeats Steps 7 and 8 until the medication has been administered over the correct amount of time.			

PROCEDURE STEPS	Yes	No	COMMENTS
12. Unclamps or releases pinching of the tubing and resets at the correct infusion rate (if the tubing was clamped during medication administration).			

Recommendation: Pass _____ Needs more practice _____

Student: _____   Date: _____

Instructor: _____   Date: _____

PROCEDURE CHECKLIST
Chapter 26: Administering IV Push Medications Through an Intermittent Device (IV Lock) When No Extension Tubing Is Attached to the Venous Access Device

Check (✓) Yes or No

PROCEDURE STEPS	Yes	No	COMMENTS
Before, during, and after the procedure, follows Principles-Based Checklist to Use With All Procedures, including: Identifies the patient according to agency policy using two identifiers; attends appropriately to standard precautions, hand hygiene, safety, privacy, body mechanics, and documentation.			
1. Checks compatibility of the medication with the existing IV solution, if one is infusing.			
2. Prepares the medication from a vial or ampule. Dilutes the medication as needed.			
3. Selects the appropriate size syringe for flush solution.			
4. Dons clean procedure gloves.			
5. Thoroughly scrubs all surfaces of the injection port closest to the patient with an alcohol prep pad or CHG-alcohol combination product.			
6. Inserts the flush syringe into the injection port.			
7. Depending on the equipment, gently aspirates for a blood return by pulling back on the plunger to check for a blood return.			
8. If blood returns when using equipment requiring aspirations, administers a flush solution to clear the line if blood return is obtained. Uses a forward pushing motion on the syringe, with a slow, steady injection technique. If no blood returns, assesses patency by administering a small amount of flush solution and monitors for ease of administration, swelling at IV site, patient complaint of discomfort at site.			
9. Continues to hold injection port, removes and recaps flush syringe using a one-handed method, then scrubs port with an alcohol prep pad or CHG-alcohol product, and attaches the medication syringe.			
10. Administers the medication in small increments over the correct time interval.			

PROCEDURE STEPS	Yes	No	COMMENTS
11. Continuing to hold injection port, removes medication syringe. Scrubs all surfaces of the port with alcohol prep pad or CHG-alcohol product. Attaches the flush syringe.			
12. Administers the flush solution.			
13. Uses positive pressure when removing the syringe by placing the thumb or index finger to avoid movement of the plunger.			

Recommendation: Pass _____ Needs more practice _____

Student: _____   Date: _____

Instructor: _____   Date: _____

PROCEDURE CHECKLIST
Chapter 26: Administering IV Push Medications Through an Intermittent Device With IV Extension Tubing

Check (✔) Yes or No

PROCEDURE STEPS	Yes	No	COMMENTS
Before, during, and after the procedure, follows Principles-Based Checklist to Use With All Procedures, including: Identifies the patient according to agency policy using two identifiers; attends appropriately to standard precautions, hand hygiene, safety, privacy, body mechanics, and documentation.			
1. Checks compatibility of medication with existing intravenous solution, if infusing.			
2. Prepares medication from vial or ampule. Dilutes as needed.			
3. Determines the volume of any extension tubing attached to the access port.			
4. Dons clean procedure gloves.			
5. Scrubs all surfaces of the injection port with an antiseptic wipe.			
6. If using a connector that requires aspiration, gently pulling back on plunger to check for blood return. If no blood returns, assesses patency by administering a small amount of the flush solution and monitoring for ease of administration, swelling at the IV site, or patient complaint of discomfort at the site. (Newer connectors may not require or allow for aspirating; follow agency policy.)			
7. Administers flush after establishing patency of the IV line.			
8. Scrubs the port. Attaches the medication syringe and injects a volume of medication equal to the volume of the extension set at the same rate as flush solution.			
9. Uses slow, steady injection technique and administers remainder of the medication over the prescribed interval for the specific medication. Does not force the flush solution.			
10. Continues to hold the injection connector and removes medication syringe.			
11. Scrubs all surfaces of the injection connector for at least 15 seconds and attaches the flush syringe.			
12. Administers the same amount of flush solution at the same rate as the medication, then administers the remainder of the flush solution.			

PROCEDURE STEPS	Yes	No	COMMENTS
13. Uses a slow, steady injection pressure technique when removing syringe. Continues to administer the flush solution while withdrawing the syringe cannula from the injection port. Follows equipment instructions regarding the method and order of removing the syringe, closing the clamp, maintaining positive pressure.			
14. Properly disposes of used equipment.			

Recommendation: Pass _____ Needs more practice _____

Student: _____   Date: _____

Instructor: _____   Date: _____

PROCEDURE CHECKLIST
Chapter 26: Administering Medication Through a Central Venous Access Device (CVAD)

Check (✓) Yes or No

PROCEDURE STEPS	Yes	No	COMMENTS
Before, during, and after the procedure, follows Principles-Based Checklist to Use With All Procedures, including: Identifies the patient according to agency policy using two identifiers; attends appropriately to standard precautions, hand hygiene, safety, privacy, body mechanics, and documentation.			
1. Prepares medications as follows:			
a. Checks compatibility of the medication with the existing IV solution, if one is infusing.			
b. Verifies the medication can safely be administered through a central site. Double-checks infusion rate.			
c. Draws up the medication using a needleless device or needle with a filter.			
d. Recaps needles throughout, using a needle capping device or approved one-handed technique that has a low risk of contaminating the sterile needle. Dilutes medication, if needed. Fills medication syringe to the exact volume to be infused, expels excess volume.			
e. Labels syringe with contents; includes medication name, dilution, time to be administered, route, name of person constituting medication.			
2. Flushes the line.			
a. Obtains heparinized or saline solution for flushing the CVAD, according to agency's policy.			
b. Before flushing the CVAD, examines the syringe for bubbles. Removes them by flicking the syringe. Ejects the bubbles but ensures there is enough flush solution remaining in the syringe.			

Copyright © 2016, F. A. Davis Company, Wilkinson & Treas/Procedure Checklists for Fundamentals of Nursing, 3e

PROCEDURE STEPS	Yes	No	COMMENTS
c. Dons clean procedure gloves. Using an antiseptic prep pad, vigorously scrubs CVAD connectors, Luer Locking threads, or Luer-Lock; includes the extension "tail." Scrubs for at least 15 seconds and allows to dry for 15 seconds (or per manufacturer's guidelines). Does not touch connector after cleansing.			
d. Inserts flush syringe at a vertical angle into the port using a needleless system or safety syringe.			
e. Opens the clamp between the syringe and patient.			
f. Checks for blood return by pulling the syringe plunger back.			
g. Clears the line by flushing or running IV fluid.			
h. Injects saline or heparinized flush solution into the line, per agency protocol or provider's prescription. Does not force flush solution into venous access device. If resistance, checks for a closed clamp on catheter or tubing, and checks to see if an inline filter is clogged.			
i. Closes clamp.			
j. Disconnects flush syringe after flushing. Because techniques of flushing and clamping vary, follow agency protocols. Uses correct technique for negative, positive, or neutral displacement devices. Uses correct technique for a blunt cannula or mechanical valve, or mechanical valve with negative displacement.			
k. Discards flush syringe in a safety disposal container, after removing from port.			
3. Administers medication through the CVAD.			
a. Scrubs the CVAD port or Luer-Lock on all sides with an approved antiseptic prep pad. Allows the port to dry for 15 more seconds (or per manufacturer's guidelines).			
b. Closes clamp to the infusion, if a primary IV is running.			
c. Slowly injects medication into the port, according to the medication order (infusion time).			
4. After scrubbing all surfaces of the port again with an approved antiseptic pad, administers the second syringe of flush solution.			

PROCEDURE STEPS	Yes	No	COMMENTS
5. Clamps the tubing between the syringe and the CVAD port, making sure it is open between the IV fluid and patient, if there is a running IV.			

Recommendation: Pass _____ Needs more practice _____

Student: _____ Date: _____

Instructor: _____ Date: _____

Copyright © 2016, F. A. Davis Company, Wilkinson & Treas/Procedure Checklists for Fundamentals of Nursing, 3e

Check (✔) Yes or No

PROCEDURE STEPS	Yes	No	COMMENTS
Before, during, and after the procedure, follows Principles-Based Checklist to Use With All Procedures, including: Identifies the patient according to agency policy using two identifiers; attends appropriately to standard precautions, hand hygiene, safety, privacy, body mechanics, and documentation.			
1. Prepares and administers medications.			

2.   Follows steps in Procedure Checklist Chapter 26: Administering Oral Medications.
    a. Gives liquid form of medication when possible. Dilutes hypertonic solutions with 10–30 mL of sterile water before instilling.
    b. Verifies tablets can be crushed and given through the enteral tube.
    c. Crushes tablets and mixes with about 20 mL of water. Gives medications separately.			

3. Dons nonsterile procedure gloves.			
4. Places patient in sitting (high Fowler's) position if possible.			
5. Checks nasogastric tube placement by aspirating stomach contents and measuring the pH of the aspirate, if possible. Other, less accurate, methods are injecting air into the feeding tube and auscultating, or asking patient to speak. Uses a combination of bedside methods.			
6. Checks for residual volume.			
7. Flushes the tube, uses the correct type and size syringe. To flush the tube, removes the bulb or plunger from the syringe, attaches barrel to the tube, and pours in 20–30 mL of water.			
8. Instills medication by depressing the syringe plunger or using the barrel of the syringe as a funnel and pouring in the medication. Smaller tubes require instilling with a 30- to 60-mL syringe; the medication can be poured with larger tubes.			
9. Flushes the medication through the tube by instilling an additional 20–30 mL of water.			

PROCEDURE STEPS	Yes	No	COMMENTS
10. If giving more than one medication, gives each separately and flushes after each.			
11. Has patient maintain a sitting position (if able) for at least 30 minutes after medication administration.			

Recommendation: Pass _____ Needs more practice _____

Student: _____   Date: _____

Instructor: _____   Date: _____

Check (✓) Yes or No

PROCEDURE STEPS	Yes	No	COMMENTS
Before, during, and after the procedure, follows Principles-Based Checklist to Use With All Procedures, including: Identifies the patient according to agency policy using two identifiers; attends appropriately to standard precautions, hand hygiene, safety, privacy, body mechanics, and documentation.			
1. Identifies the amount of medication for inhalation remaining in the canister. Based on the start date and instructions for use, determines the number of remaining inhalations. Replaces the canister promptly when the canister is nearly empty.			
2. Assists patient to a seated position.			
3. Asks patient to rinse out his mouth and to spit the fluid out (not swallow).			
4. Shakes the inhaler. Removes the mouthpiece cap of the inhaler and inserts the mouthpiece into the spacer while holding the canister upright.			
5. Removes the cap from the spacer.			
6. Asks patient to breathe out slowly and completely.			
7. Places the spacer mouthpiece into patient's mouth and has him seal his lips around the mouthpiece. Sharply presses down on the inhaler canister to discharge one puff of medication into the spacer.			
8. Asks patients to slowly inhale and then hold his breath for as long as possible. Encourages patient to hold his breath for 10 seconds if possible.			
9. If a second puff is needed, waits at least 1 minute before repeating Steps 6 through 8.			
10. If a corticosteroid inhaler was used, assists patient to rinse out his mouth with water and spit out the rinse.			
11. Wipes the mouthpiece with a tissue or moist cloth and replaces the cap. Periodically rinses the spacer, mouthpiece, and cap with water.			

PROCEDURE STEPS	Yes	No	COMMENTS

Recommendation: Pass _____ Needs more practice _____

Student: _____   Date: _____

Instructor: _____   Date: _____

PROCEDURE CHECKLIST
Chapter 26: Administering Nasal Medication

Check (✓) Yes or No

PROCEDURE STEPS	Yes	No	COMMENTS
Before, during, and after the procedure, follows Principles-Based Checklist to Use With All Procedures, including: Identifies the patient according to agency policy using two identifiers; attends appropriately to standard precautions, hand hygiene, safety, privacy, body mechanics, and documentation.			
1. Explains to patient medication may have an unusual taste or cause some burning or tingling.			
2. Asks patient to blow his nose.			
3. Dons clean procedure gloves.			
4. Determines head position. Considers indication for medication and patient's ability to assume position. Positions patient: a. Nose drops or spray: To get head down and forward, assists patient to sit and lean forward or kneel on the bed with head dependent.			
b. To medicate ethmoid and sphenoid sinuses, assists patient into the supine position with head over the edge of the bed. Supports head. Alternatively, places a towel roll behind shoulders, allowing head to drop back.			
c. To medicate frontal and maxillary sinuses, positions as in Step 4b, but tilts the head toward affected side.			
d. If patient is unable to assume one of those positions, asks patient to tilt his head back.			
5. Asks patient to exhale and close one nostril.			
6. Administers spray or drops while patient is inhaling through nose. Does not touch dropper to sides of nostril.			
7. Repeats Steps 5 and 6 on other nostril.			
8. If nose drops are used, asks patient to stay in same position for 1–5 minutes (follows manufacturer's guidelines).			
9. Instructs patient not to blow his nose for several minutes.			

Recommendation: Pass _____ Needs more practice _____

Student: _____   Date: _____

Instructor: _____   Date: _____

PROCEDURE CHECKLIST
Chapter 26: Administering Ophthalmic Medications

Check (✓) Yes or No

PROCEDURE STEPS	Yes	No	COMMENTS
Before, during, and after the procedure, follows Principles-Based Checklist to Use With All Procedures, including: Identifies the patient according to agency policy using two identifiers; attends appropriately to standard precautions, hand hygiene, safety, privacy, body mechanics, and documentation.			
1. Assists patient to a high Fowler's position with head slightly tilted back.			
2. Dons clean procedure gloves.			
3. Cleans edges of eyelid from inner to outer canthus.			
Instilling Eye Drops:			
4. Holding the eyedropper, rests the dominant hand on patient's forehead.			
5. With the nondominant hand, pulls the lower lid down to expose the conjunctival sac.			
6. Positions eyedropper 1.5–2.0 cm (½ ¾ in.) above patient's eye; does not let the dropper touch the eye. Asks patient to look up; drops the correct number of drops into the conjunctival sac. Does not drop onto cornea.			
7. Asks patient to gently close eyes.			
8. If the medication has systemic effects, presses gently against the same side of the nose to close the lacrimal ducts for 1–2 minutes.			
Administering Eye Ointment:			
9. Rests the dominant hand, with eye ointment, on patient's forehead.			
10. With the nondominant hand, pulls the lower lid down to expose the conjunctival sac.			
11. Asks patient to look up.			
12. Applies a thin strip of ointment (about 1 in. [2–2.5 cm]) in conjunctival sac; twists wrist to break off the strip of ointment.			
13. Does not let the tube touch the eye.			
14. Asks patient to gently close eyes for 2–3 minutes. Alternatively, has the patient blink several times.			

PROCEDURE STEPS	Yes	No	COMMENTS
15. Explains to patient that vision will be blurred for a short time.			

<u>Recommendation</u>: Pass _____ Needs more practice _____

Student: _____   Date: _____

Instructor: _____   Date: _____

PROCEDURE CHECKLIST
Chapter 26: Administering Oral Medications

Check (✓) Yes or No

PROCEDURE STEPS	Yes	No	COMMENTS
Before, during, and after the procedure, follows Principles-Based Checklist to Use With All Procedures, including: Identifies the patient according to agency policy using two identifiers; attends appropriately to standard precautions, hand hygiene, safety, privacy, body mechanics, and documentation.			
1. Prepares and administers medications.			
Variation. Tablets and Capsules:			
2. If pouring from a multidose container, does not touch the medication. Pours the tablet into the cap of the bottle, then into the medication cup.			
3. Pours the correct number of tablets into the medication cup.			
4. If necessary to give less than a whole tablet, breaks a scored tablet with gloved hands; uses a pill cutter if necessary. Does not break an unscored tablet.			
5. If the drug is unit-dose, does not open package; places entire package in paper (soufflé) cup.			
6. If patient has difficulty swallowing, checks to see if tablet can be crushed. If so, mixes with soft food.			
7. Pours all medications scheduled at the same time into same cup, except uses a separate cup for any medications requiring preadministration assessment.			
8. Completes preadministration assessments if needed.			
9. If patient is able to hold it, places tablet or medication cup in her hand. If unable to hold it, places medication cup to her lips and tips tablet(s) into her mouth.			
10. Provides a liquid to swallow tablets.			
Variation. Sublingual Medications:			
11. Places, or asks patient to place the tablet under the tongue and hold there until completely dissolved.			
Variation. Buccal Medications:			
12. Places, or asks patient to place, the tablet between the cheek and gums and hold there until completely dissolved.			

Copyright © 2016, F. A. Davis Company, Wilkinson & Treas/Procedure Checklists for Fundamentals of Nursing, 3e

PROCEDURE STEPS	Yes	No	COMMENTS
Variation. Liquids:			
13. Shakes the liquid, if necessary, before opening the container.			
14. Places the bottle with lid flat side down on the counter.			
15. Holds the bottle with the label in the palm of the hand.			
16. Pours the medication, and slightly twists the bottle when finished to prevent dripping.			
17. If medication drips over bottle lip when pouring, wipes with a clean tissue or paper towel—only the outside lip of the bottle.			
18. Holds the medication cup at eye level to measure the dosage.			
19. Positions patient in a sitting (high Fowler's) position if possible; or raises the head of the bed as much as allowed.			

Recommendation: Pass _____ Needs more practice _____

Student: _____ Date: _____

Instructor: _____ Date: _____

PROCEDURE CHECKLIST
Chapter 26: Administering Otic Medications

Check (✓) Yes or No

PROCEDURE STEPS	Yes	No	COMMENTS
Before, during, and after the procedure, follows Principles-Based Checklist to Use With All Procedures, including: Identifies the patient according to agency policy using two identifiers; attends appropriately to standard precautions, hand hygiene, safety, privacy, body mechanics, and documentation.			
1. Warms the solution to be instilled (e.g., in hand or in warm, not hot, water) and gently shakes the bottle before using the drops.			
2. Assists patient to a side-lying position, or turn patient's head to the side, with the appropriate ear facing up.			
3. Cleans the external ear with a cotton-tipped applicator if needed.			
4. Fills the dropper with the correct amount of medication.			
5. For infants and young children, asks another caregiver to immobilize the child while administering the medication.			
6 Straightens the ear canal. a. For patients 3 years and older, pulls pinna upward and back.			
b. For children younger than 3 years old, pulls pinna down and back.			
7. Instills correct number of drops along the side of the ear canal.			
8. Does not touch the end of the dropper to any part of the ear.			
9. Gently tugs on the external ear after drops are instilled.			
10. Instructs patient to keep her head turned to the side for 5–10 minutes.			
11. Places cotton loosely at the opening of the auditory canal for 15 minutes.			

Recommendation: Pass _____ Needs more practice _____

Student: _____   Date: _____

Instructor: _____   Date: _____

Copyright © 2016, F. A. Davis Company, Wilkinson & Treas/Procedure Checklists for Fundamentals of Nursing, 3e

PROCEDURE CHECKLIST
Chapter 26: Administering Subcutaneous Medications

Check (✔) Yes or No

PROCEDURE STEPS	Yes	No	COMMENTS
Before, during, and after the procedure, follows Principles-Based Checklist to Use With All Procedures, including: Identifies the patient according to agency policy using two identifiers; attends appropriately to standard precautions, hand hygiene, safety, privacy, body mechanics, and documentation.			
1. Selects appropriate syringe and needle. Considers amount of adipose tissue: a. For insulin, must use an insulin syringe—typically 0.3, 0.5, or 1.0 mL. Most insulin needles are 28–31-gauge. Needle length is often $\frac{3}{16}$–1 inch.			
b. For non-insulin volumes less than 1 ml, uses a tuberculin (TB) syringe with a 25–27-gauge, $\frac{3}{8}$–$\frac{5}{8}$-inch needle.			
c. For a non-insulin volume of 1 mL, a 3-mL syringe may be used with a 25–27 gauge, $\frac{3}{8}$–$\frac{5}{8}$-inch needle.			
2. Draws up medication. See checklist for Preparing and Drawing Up Medication: Mixing Medications From Two Vials. Does not give more than 1 mL of medication in a site.			
3. Selects appropriate site (outer aspect of the upper arms, abdomen, anterior aspects of the thighs, high on buttocks near waist level, and the scapular area on upper back). The site must have adequate subcutaneous tissue. For heparin, abdomen is the only site used.			
4. Positions patient so injection site is accessible and patient can relax the muscle.			
5. Dons clean procedure gloves.			
6. Scrubs injection site with an antiseptic pad by circling from center of the site outward (for alcohol) or using a back-and-forth motion (for CHG products). Does not move back over already cleaned tissue. Allows site to dry before administering the injection.			
7. Removes needle cap.			

PROCEDURE STEPS	Yes	No	COMMENTS
8. With the nondominant hand, pinches or pulls taut the skin at the injection site.			
a. If patient is obese or "pinch" of adipose tissue is greater than 2 in., uses a 90° angle.			
b. If patient is average size or "pinch" is less than 1 in., uses a 45° angle.			
c. If patient is obese and the adipose tissue pinches 2 in. or more, uses a longer needle (if available) and spreads skin taut instead of pinching. Enters tissue at a 90° angle.			
9. Holds the syringe between thumb and index finger of the dominant hand like a pencil or dart, and inserts the needle at the appropriate angle into the pinched-up skinfold (spreads skin taut in obese patients).			
10. Stabilizes the syringe with the fingers of the nondominant hand.			
11. Using the thumb or index finger of the dominant hand, presses the plunger slowly to inject the medication. (Alternatively, after inserting the needle, continues to hold the barrel with the dominant hand and uses the nondominant hand to depress the plunger.) Does not give more than 1 mL of medication in a site.			
12. Removes the safety needle smoothly along the line of insertion.			
13. Gently blots any blood with a gauze pad.			
14. Engages the needle safety device or places the uncapped syringe and needle directly into a sharps container.			

Recommendation: Pass _____ Needs more practice _____

Student: _____ Date: _____

Instructor: _____ Date: _____

PROCEDURE CHECKLIST
Chapter 26: Administering Vaginal Medications

Check (✓) Yes or No

PROCEDURE STEPS	Yes	No	COMMENTS
For All Vaginal Medications:			
Before, during, and after the procedure, follows Principles-Based Checklist to Use With All Procedures, including: Identifies the patient according to agency policy using two identifiers; attends appropriately to standard precautions, hand hygiene, safety, privacy, body mechanics, and documentation.			
1. Prepares and administers medication.			
2. Asks patient to void before the procedure.			
3. Positions patient in a dorsal recumbent or Sims' position.			
4. Drapes patient with a bath blanket with only the perineum exposed.			
5. Prepares medication: a. Removes wrapper from the suppository and places loosely in wrapper container.			
b. Or fills applicator according to the manufacturer's instructions.			
6. For irrigations, uses warm solution (temperature approximately 105°F [40.6°C]).			
7. Uses only water-soluble lubricant.			
8. Inspects and cleans around vaginal orifice.			
Administering a Suppository:			
9. Dons clean procedure gloves; applies a water-soluble lubricant to the rounded end of the suppository and to the gloved index finger on the dominant hand.			
10. Separates the labia with the gloved nondominant hand.			
11. Inserts suppository as far as possible along the posterior vaginal wall (about 3 in. [8 cm]). If the suppository comes with an applicator, places the suppository in the end of the applicator, inserts the applicator into the vagina, and presses the plunger.			
12. Asks patient to remain in a supine position for 5–15 minutes. May elevate her hips on a pillow.			

PROCEDURE STEPS	Yes	No	COMMENTS
Applicator Insertion of Cream, Foam, or Jelly:			
13. Separates the labia with nondominant hand.			
14. Inserts the applicator approximately 3 in. (8 cm) into vagina along the posterior vaginal wall.			
15. Depresses the plunger, emptying medication into the vagina.			
16. Disposes of the applicator or places on paper towel if reusable; cleanses later.			
17. Asks patient to remain supine for 5–15 minutes.			
Vaginal Irrigation:			
18. Hangs irrigation solution approximately 1–2 feet (30–60 cm) above level of patient's vagina.			
19. Assists patient into a dorsal recumbent position.			
20. Places a waterproof pad and bedpan under patient.			
21. If using a vaginal irrigation set with tubing, opens the clamp to allow the solution to fill the tubing completely.			
22. Lubricates end of the irrigation nozzle.			
23. Inserts nozzle approximately 3 in. (7–8 cm) into the vagina, directing it toward the sacrum.			
24. Starts the flow of the irrigation solution, and rotates nozzle intermittently as solution is flowing.			
25. If labia are reddened, runs some of the solution over the labia.			
26. After all irrigating solution has been used, removes the nozzle and assists patient to a sitting position on the bedpan (to drain the solution).			
27. Removes bedpan.			
28. Cleanses perineum with toilet tissue or perineal wash solution and washcloth or wipes. Dries perineum.			
29. Applies perineal pad if excessive drainage.			

Recommendation: Pass _____ Needs more practice _____

Student: _____   Date: _____

Instructor: _____   Date: _____

PROCEDURE CHECKLIST
Chapter 26: Applying Medications to the Skin

Check (✓) Yes or No

PROCEDURE STEPS	Yes	No	COMMENTS
Before, during, and after the procedure, follows Principles-Based Checklist to Use With All Procedures, including: Identifies the patient according to agency policy using two identifiers; attends appropriately to standard precautions, hand hygiene, safety, privacy, body mechanics, and documentation.			
Lotions, Creams, and Ointments:			
1. Dons clean gloves.			
2. Cleanses skin with wipes or soap and water, per agency policy. Pats dry before applying to enhance absorption.			
3. Warms medication in gloved hands.			
4. Uses gloves or an applicator to apply and spread the medication evenly, following the direction of hair growth when coating the area.			
Topical Aerosol Sprays:			
1. Dons clean gloves.			
2. Cleanses skin with cleansing wipe or soap and water (according to agency policy). Pats dry before applying to enhance absorption.			
3. Shakes container to mix the contents.			
4. Holds container at the distance specified on the label (usually 6–12 in.) and sprays over the prescribed area. (Usually, holds upright.)			
5. If spraying near patient's head, covers face with towel.			
Powders:			
1. Dons clean gloves.			
2. Cleanses skin with cleansing wipe or soap and water (according to agency policy), and pats dry before applying to enhance absorption.			
3. Spreads apart skinfolds and applies a very thin layer.			
4. Applies the powder to clean, dry skin. Is careful that patient does not inhale the powder.			

PROCEDURE STEPS	Yes	No	COMMENTS
Transdermal Medications:			
1. Dons clean gloves.			
2. Removes the previous patch, folds the medicated side to the inside.			
3. Disposes of the old patch carefully in an appropriate receptacle.			
4. Cleanses skin, removes any remaining medication. Allows skin to dry.			
5. Removes patch from its protective covering, and removes the clear, protective covering without touching the adhesive or the inside surface that contains the medication.			
6. Applies patch to a clean, dry, hairless (or little hair), intact skin area. Presses down on patch for about 10 seconds with the palm. Does not use areas with lesions or irritation.			
7. Rotates application sites. Common sites are trunk, lower abdomen, lower back, buttocks.			
8. Teaches patient to not use a heating pad over area.			
9. Writes date, time, initials on new patch.			
10. Removes gloves, performs hand hygiene.			
11. Observes for local side effects (such as skin irritation, itching, and allergic contact dermatitis).			
12. For medications packaged in ointment form and applied on calibrated paper, wears gloves; applies ointment in a continuous motion along those marks to measure the required dose. Folds paper in half to distribute the ointment evenly on the patch.			

Recommendation: Pass _____ Needs more practice _____

Student: _____   Date: _____

Instructor: _____   Date: _____

PROCEDURE CHECKLIST
Chapter 26: Inserting a Rectal Suppository

Check (✓) Yes or No

PROCEDURE STEPS	Yes	No	COMMENTS
Before, during, and after the procedure, follows Principles-Based Checklist to Use With All Procedures, including: Identifies the patient according to agency policy using two identifiers; attends appropriately to standard precautions, hand hygiene, safety, privacy, body mechanics, and documentation.			
1. Prepares and administers medication.			
2. Asks patient if he needs to defecate prior to suppository insertion.			
3. Assists patient to Sims' position.			
4. Dons clean procedure gloves.			
5. If patient is uncooperative (e.g., confused, child), obtains help to immobilize patient while inserting suppository.			
6. Removes suppository wrapper and lubricates smooth end of the suppository and tip of the gloved index finger.			
7. Explains there will be a cool feeling from the lubricant and a feeling of pressure during insertion.			
8. Uses nondominant hand to separate buttocks.			
9. Asks patient to take deep breaths in and out through the mouth.			
10. Uses index finger of the dominant hand to gently insert suppository, lubricated smooth end first; or follows manufacturer's instructions.			
11. Does not force the suppository during insertion.			
12. Pushes the suppository past the internal sphincter and along the rectal wall (about 1–3 in. [5 cm] in an adult; ½–1 in. [2 cm] for an infant).			
13. Asks patient to retain the suppository if able. If he has difficulty retaining suppository, after removing finger from anus, holds buttocks together for several seconds.			
14. Wipes anus with toilet tissue.			

PROCEDURE STEPS	Yes	No	COMMENTS
15. Explains to patient the need to remain in side-lying position for 5–10 minutes.			
16. Disposes used materials into a biohazard receptacle; washes hands thoroughly.			
17. Leaves call light and bedpan within patient's reach if suppository was a laxative.			

Recommendation: Pass _____ Needs more practice _____

Student: _____   Date: _____

Instructor: _____   Date: _____

PROCEDURE CHECKLIST
Chapter 26: Irrigating the Eyes

Check (✓) Yes or No

PROCEDURE STEPS	Yes	No	COMMENTS
Before, during, and after the procedure, follows Principles-Based Checklist to Use With All Procedures, including: Identifies the patient according to agency policy using two identifiers; attends appropriately to standard precautions, hand hygiene, safety, privacy, body mechanics, and documentation.			
1. Assists patient to a low-Fowler's position (if possible), with head tilted toward affected eye.			
2. Places a towel and basin under patient's cheek.			
3. Checks pH by gently touching pH paper to secretions in the conjunctival sac (normal is approximately 7.1).			
4. Instills ocular anesthetic drops, if ordered. Follows agency protocol.			
5. Connects IV solution and tubing; primes the tubing.			
6. Holds IV tubing about 1 inch (2.5 cm) from the eye; does not touch the eye.			
7. Separates eyelids with thumb and index finger.			
8. Directs flow of the solution over the eye from inner to outer canthus.			
9. Rechecks pH and continues to irrigate the eye as needed.			

Recommendation: Pass _____ Needs more practice _____

Student: _____   Date: _____

Instructor: _____   Date: _____

Copyright © 2016, F. A. Davis Company, Wilkinson & Treas/Procedure Checklists for Fundamentals of Nursing, 3e

Check (✓) Yes or No

PROCEDURE STEPS	Yes	No	COMMENTS
Before, during, and after the procedure, follows Principles-Based Checklist to Use With All Procedures, including: Identifies the patient according to agency policy using two identifiers; attends appropriately to standard precautions, hand hygiene, safety, privacy, body mechanics, and documentation.			
1. Palpates landmarks and muscle mass to ensure correct location and muscle adequacy.			
Deltoid Site:			
1. Uses site for small amounts of medication, immunizations, or when ventrogluteal or vastus lateralis sites are contraindicated.			
2. Completely exposes patient's upper arm; removes garment if necessary.			
3. Locates lower edge of acromion (which forms the base of a triangle).			
4. Draws imaginary line from each end of the triangle base downward 1 to 2 in. (3 to 5 cm) to the midpoint of the lateral arm. The resulting inverted triangle is the deltoid site.			
5. An alternative approach is to place four fingerbreadths across the deltoid muscle with the top finger on the acromion process. The injection goes three fingerbreadths below the process.			
Rectus Femoris:			
(Not a site of choice)			
1. Divides top of thigh from groin to knee into thirds and identifies the middle third. Visualizes a rectangle in the middle of the anterior surface of the thigh. This is the location of the injection site.			
Vastus Lateralis:			
1. Instructs patient to assume a supine or sitting position.			
2. Locates greater trochanter and the lateral femoral condyle.			
3. Places hands on patient's thigh with one hand against the greater trochanter and edge of the other hand against the lateral femoral condyle.			

Copyright © 2016, F. A. Davis Company, Wilkinson & Treas/Procedure Checklists for Fundamentals of Nursing, 3e

PROCEDURE STEPS	Yes	No	COMMENTS
4. Visualizes a rectangle between the hands across the anterolateral thigh. • The index fingers of the hands form the smaller ends of the rectangle. • The long sides of the rectangle are formed by (a) drawing an imaginary line down the center of the anterior thigh and (b) drawing another line along the side of the leg, halfway between the bed and the front of the thigh. • This box marks the middle third of the anterolateral thigh, which is the injection site.			
Ventrogluteal Site:			
1. Instructs patient to assume a side-lying position, if possible.			
2. Locates greater trochanter, anterior superior iliac spine, and iliac crest.			
3. Places palm of hand on greater trochanter, index finger on anterior superior iliac spine, and middle finger pointing toward the iliac crest. (Uses the right hand on patient's left hip; uses the left hand on patient's right hip.)			
4. The middle of the triangle between the middle and index fingers is the injection site.			

Recommendation: Pass _____ Needs more practice _____

Student: _____   Date: _____

Instructor: _____   Date: _____   .

Check (✓) Yes or No

PROCEDURE STEPS	Yes	No	COMMENTS
Before, during, and after the procedure, follows Principles-Based Checklist to Use With All Procedures, including: Identifies the patient according to agency policy using two identifiers; attends appropriately to standard precautions, hand hygiene, safety, privacy, body mechanics, and documentation.			
Refers to Procedure Checklist for Drawing Up Medications From Ampules for handling ampules; Drawing Up Medications From Vials; and Clinical Insight: Measuring Dosages When Changing Needles in Volume 1.			
1. Checks compatibility of medications.			
2. With filter needle (or cannula), withdraws exact amount of medication. Ejects air bubbles (keeping syringe vertical) and excess air as needed to obtain correct dose.			
3. Pulls back on plunger to withdraw all medication from needle (or filter cannula or vial access device) into syringe. Depending on size of the access device, this may be as much as 0.2 mL. It will appear there is more than the ordered dose in the syringe.			
4. Changes to the needle to be used for injection.			
5. Holds the syringe vertically, and ejects air until nurse sees a drop of medication at the tip of the needle ("drop to the top").			
6. Measures the medication. Verifies at the correct syringe marking. If not, tips the syringe horizontally and ejects the medication until the dose is correct.			
7. Injects patient with the correct dose. Some medication will remain in the needle.			
8. If giving an irritating medication (e.g., iron), draws 0.2 mL of air into the syringe before giving the injection. Follows procedure for administering an air lock injection.			

Copyright © 2016, F. A. Davis Company, Wilkinson & Treas/Procedure Checklists for Fundamentals of Nursing, 3e

PROCEDURES STEPS	Yes	No	COMMENTS

Recommendation: Pass _____ Needs more practice _____

Student: _____   Date: _____

Instructor: _____   Date: _____

PROCEDURE CHECKLIST
Chapter 26: Drawing Up Medications From Ampules

Check (✓) Yes or No

PROCEDURE STEPS	Yes	No	COMMENTS
Before, during, and after the procedure, follows Principles-Based Checklist to Use With All Procedures, including: Identifies the patient according to agency policy using two identifiers; attends appropriately to standard precautions, hand hygiene, safety, privacy, body mechanics, and documentation.			
1. Flicks or taps the top of the ampule to remove medication trapped in the top of the ampule. Alternatively, shakes the ampule by quickly turning and "snapping" the wrist.			
2. Uses ampule snapper, or wraps 2 in. × 2 in. gauze pad or unwrapped antiseptic pad around neck of the ampule; using dominant hand, snaps off the top, breaking the ampule top away from the body.			
3. Attaches filter needle (or filter straw) to a syringe. If the syringe has a needle in place, removes both the needle and the cap and places on a sterile surface (e.g., a newly unwrapped antiseptic pad still in the open wrapper), then attaches filter needle.			
4. Uses one of the following techniques to withdraw medication. Does not touch the neck of the ampule with the filter needle or filter straw: a. Inverts ampule, places needle or straw tip in liquid, and withdraws all of the medication. Does not insert the needle through the medication into the air at the top of the inverted ampule.			
b. Alternatively, tips the ampule, places the needle or access device in liquid, withdraws all of the medication. Repositions the ampule with tip remaining in the liquid.			
5. Holds syringe vertically and draws 0.2 mL of air into syringe. Measures the exact medication dose (draws back plunger to the "dose + 0.2 mL" line).			
6. Removes the filter needle or straw and reattaches the "saved" (or other sterile) needle for administration.			
7. Ejects 0.2 mL of air, and checks the dose again.			
(If giving an irritating medication such as parenteral iron, omits this step.)			

PROCEDURE STEPS	Yes	No	COMMENTS
8. Disposes top and bottom of ampule and filter needle in a sharps container.			
9. If recapping is needed, recaps needles throughout, using needle capping device or approved one-handed technique that has a low risk of contaminating the sterile needle (see Procedure Checklist, Recapping Needles Using One-Handed Technique).			

Recommendation: Pass _____ Needs more practice _____

Student: _____   Date: _____

Instructor: _____   Date: _____

PROCEDURE CHECKLIST
Chapter 26: Mixing Medications From One Ampule and Vial

Check (✓) Yes or No

PROCEDURE STEPS	Yes	No	COMMENTS
Before, during, and after the procedure, follows Principles-Based Checklist to Use With All Procedures, including: Identifies the patient according to agency policy using two identifiers; attends appropriately to standard precautions, hand hygiene, safety, privacy, body mechanics, and documentation.			
1. Begins with vial and scrubs stopper of multidose vial using an antiseptic prep pad.			
2. Attaches a vial access device (VAD) and draws up same volume of air as the dose of medication ordered for the vial.			
3. Keeps tip of the safety needle (or VAD) above the medication, injects the amount of air equal to the volume of drug to be withdrawn from the vial.			
4. Inverts vial and withdraws the prescribed volume of medication, keeping the VAD tip in the fluid.			
5. Expels any air bubbles, measures dose at eye level. Rechecks dosage, and withdraws more or ejects drug as needed.			
6. Safely recaps and removes safety needle or VAD from the syringe. Places on an opened, sterile alcohol wipe.			
7. Attaches filter needle or filter straw to syringe. (Next, draws medication from ampule.)			
8. Flicks or taps top of the ampule (or snaps wrist) to remove medication from the neck of the ampule.			
9. Opens ampule by wrapping the neck of the ampule with a folded gauze pad or unopened antiseptic prep pad or uses an ampule snapper. Snaps away from body.			
10. Withdraws exact prescribed amount of medication from ampule into syringe. Draws up second medication; if total amount of two medications is incorrect, discards syringe contents and starts over.			
11. Draws 0.2 mL of air into syringe. Confirms dose is correct by holding syringe vertically and checks the dose at eye level.			

Copyright © 2016, F. A. Davis Company, Wilkinson & Treas/Procedure Checklists for Fundamentals of Nursing, 3e

PROCEDURE STEPS	Yes	No	COMMENTS
12. Recaps filter needle or straw using a needle capping device or the one-handed technique. Draws up second medication (from ampule); does not draw excess medication into syringe. If this occurs, recognizes error, discards, and repeats procedure.			
13. Removes filter needle or straw, discards in sharps container. Replaces with a new sterile safety needle for giving medication to patient.			
14. Then ejects 0.2 mL of air, checks for the correct dose. If there is excess medication in the syringe, discards and starts over.			
15. Discards used needles and ampules in a puncture-proof sharps container.			

Recommendation: Pass _____ Needs more practice _____

Student: _____ Date: _____

Instructor: _____ Date: _____

PROCEDURE CHECKLIST
Chapter26: Preparing and Drawing Up Medication: Mixing Medications
From Two Vials

Check (✓) Yes or No

PROCEDURE STEPS	Yes	No	COMMENTS
Before, during, and after the procedure, follows Principles-Based Checklist to Use With All Procedures, including: Identifies the patient according to agency policy using two identifiers; attends appropriately to standard precautions, hand hygiene, safety, privacy, body mechanics, and documentation.			
1. Scrubs tops of both vials with an antiseptic prep pad.			
2. Draws air into syringe in same amount as total medication doses for both vials.			
3. Maintaining sterility, inserts needle or vial access device (VAD) into vial in the middle of the rubber top of the vial with bevel up at a 45°–60° angle. While pushing the needle or VAD into the rubber top, gradually brings needle upright to a 90° angle.			
4. Keeping tip of needle (or vial access device) above the medication, injects amount of air equal to the volume of drug to be withdrawn from the first vial. Injects rest of air into second vial. Prevents coring.			
5. Without removing needle (or VAD) from second vial, inverts vial and withdraws ordered amount of medication. Expels air bubbles, measures dose. Removes VAD from vial, pulls back on plunger enough to pull all medications out of the VAD into syringe. Tips syringe horizontally if any medication needs to be ejected.			
6. Inserts needle or VAD into first vial, inverts and withdraws the exact ordered amount of medication, holds syringe vertical. Plunger should be at the line for the total combined dose for both vials. Does not withdraw excess medication, keeps index finger or thumb on the flange of syringe and prevents force-back by pressure. If occurs, discards medication in syringe and starts over.			
7. Recap the access needle using a needle capping device or one-handed scoop method.			
8. Places new sterile safety needle on syringe for the injection.			

PROCEDURE STEPS	Yes	No	COMMENTS
9. Holds needle vertically, expels all air, and rechecks dosage.			
10. If using a filter needle or VAD, refers to the Clinical Insight in your book, Measuring Dosage When Changing Needles.			

Recommendation: Pass _____ Needs more practice _____

Student: _____   Date: _____

Instructor: _____   Date: _____

PROCEDURE CHECKLIST
Chapter 26: Using a Prefilled Cartridge and
Single-Dose Vial—For Intravenous Administration

Check (✔) Yes or No

PROCEDURE STEPS	Yes	No	COMMENTS
Before, during, and after the procedure, follows Principles-Based Checklist to Use With All Procedures, including: Identifies patient according to agency policy using two identifiers; attends appropriately to standard precautions, hand hygiene, safety, privacy, body mechanics, and documentation.			
1. Refer to Procedure Checklists Chapter 26: Drawing Up Medications From Ampules, for handling ampules; Drawing Up Medications From Vials, for handling vials; Measuring Dosage When Changing Needles (Filter Needle).			
2. Checks compatibility of medications.			
3. Scrubs the top rubber stopper of the vial with an antiseptic prep pad.			
4. Assembles prefilled cartridge and holder.			
5. Removes needle cap from the prefilled cartridge, expels air, measures correct dose of medication.			
6. Holds cartridge with needle up, withdraws an amount of air equal to the volume of medication needed from the vial.			
7. Continues to hold syringe with needle straight up (vertically). Inserts needle into inverted vial, with the tip of the needle in the air above medication, and injects air into vial. Maintains pressure on plunger so air and/or medication does not flow back into syringe.			

8. Maintaining sterility, inserts needle or needleless device into vial without coring:
  a. Places the tip of the needle or needleless device in the middle of the rubber stopper of the vial with bevel up at a 45°–60° angle.
  b. Maintains pressure on plunger, pulls needle down into fluid. Withdraws ordered amount of vial medication. Does not withdraw any excess.			

PROCEDURE STEPS	Yes	No	COMMENTS
9. Pressure generally pushes a little less medication than needed. Withdraws amount needed for correct dose. Does not withdraw any excess.			
10. Recaps needle (uses one-handed method). If possible, removes needle from prefilled syringe and replaces with an injection cannula for IV administration. For IM injection, if prefilled syringe does not have a safety needle, transfers medication to new syringe and needle for injection.			

Recommendation: Pass _____ Needs more practice _____

Student: _____ Date: _____

Instructor: _____ Date: _____

PROCEDURE CHECKLIST
Chapter 26: Drawing Up Medications From Vials

Check (✔) Yes or No

PROCEDURE STEPS	Yes	No	COMMENTS
Before, during, and after the procedure, follows Principles-Based Checklist to Use With All Procedures, including: Identifies the patient according to agency policy using two identifiers; attends appropriately to standard precautions, hand hygiene, safety, privacy, body mechanics, and documentation.			
1. Mixes solution in vial; gently rolls vial between hands if necessary.			
2. Places vial on a flat work surface and thoroughly scrubs rubber stopper of vial with an antiseptic prep pad.			
3. Removes needle (if one is attached to the syringe). Attaches VAD and removes cap. Does not touch needle or VAD shaft.			
4. Places needle or VAD cap on a clean surface, or holds the cap open-side out between two fingers of nondominant hand.			
5. Draws air into syringe equal to the amount of medication to be withdrawn from vial.			
6. Inserts needle or vial access device (VAD) into vial without coring while maintaining sterile technique.			
a. Places tip of needle or vial access device in the middle of the rubber stopper of the vial with bevel up at a 45°–60° angle.			
b. While pushing needle or VAD into rubber stopper, gradually brings needle upright to a 90° angle.			
7. With tip of needle or VAD above fluid line, injects air in syringe, into the air in the vial.			
8. Inverts vial, keeps needle or VAD in the vial, slowly withdraws medication.			
9. Keeps needle or VAD in vial, removes any air from syringe.			
a. Carefully stabilizes vial and syringe, firmly taps syringe below the air bubbles.			
b. When air bubbles are at the hub of syringe, makes sure syringe is vertical (straight up and down), and pushes air back into vial.			
c. Withdraws additional medication if necessary to obtain correct dose.			

PROCEDURE STEPS	Yes	No	COMMENTS
10. When dose is correct, withdraws needle or VAD from vial at a 90° angle.			
11. Holds syringe upright at eye level, rechecks medication dose.			
12. Recaps VAD using a needle recapping device or the one-handed method.			
13. Before removing VAD or access needle, draws back on syringe plunger and removes all medication from dead space inVAD/needle.			
14. Removes VAD/needle, attaches the "saved" sterile needle for injection. Holds syringe vertically, expels air, if necessary. Holds syringe horizontally to expel medication.			
15. Disposes of vial and filter needles in sharps container.			

<u>Recommendation:</u> Pass _____ Needs more practice _____

Student: _____   Date: _____

Instructor: _____   Date: _____

PROCEDURE CHECKLIST
Chapter 26: Recapping Needles Using One-Handed Technique

Check (✓) Yes or No

PROCEDURE STEPS	Yes	No	COMMENTS
Before, during, and after the procedure, follows Principles-Based Checklist to Use With All Procedures, including: Identifies the patient according to agency policy using two identifiers; attends appropriately to standard precautions, hand hygiene, safety, privacy, body mechanics, and documentation.			
Recapping Contaminated Needles:			
1. If using safety needle, engages safety mechanism to cover needle.			
2. Alternatively, places needle cap in mechanical recapping device.			
3. If mechanical recapping device is not available, uses one-handed scoop method to recap the needle. a. Places needle cover on flat surface.			
b. Holds syringe in dominant hand, scoops needle cap onto needle. Tips syringe vertically to slip cover over needle. Does not hold onto needle cap with nondominant hand while scooping.			
c. Secures needle cap by grasping it near hub.			
Recapping Sterile Needles:			
1. Places needle cap in a mechanical recapping device, if available.			
Alternative method: Places cap into small liquid medication cup with open end facing up. Inserts sterile needle into cap, keeping the free hand well away from the cup.			
3. Alternative method: Places cap on clean surface so end of needle cap protrudes over edge of counter or shelf, scoops with needle; keeps free hand well away from needle and cap, as recapping.			
4. Alternative method: If syringe is packaged in a hard plastic tubular container, stands container on large end, inverts needle cap, places it in the top of the hard container. Inserts needle downward into cap.			

PROCEDURE STEPS	Yes	No	COMMENTS
5. Alternative method: Places cap on a sterile surface, such as on an open antiseptic prep pad, uses one-handed scoop technique. Does not touch anything with needle other than the inside of the needle cap.			

Recommendation: Pass _____ Needs more practice _____

Student: _____ Date: _____

Instructor: _____ Date: _____

PROCEDURE CHECKLIST
Chapter 26: Using a Piggyback Administration Set With a Gravity Infusion

Check (✔) Yes or No

PROCEDURE STEPS	Yes	No	COMMENTS
Before, during, and after the procedure, follows Principles-Based Checklist to Use With All Procedures, including: Identifies the patient according to agency policy using two identifiers; attends appropriately to standard precautions, hand hygiene, safety, privacy, body mechanics, and documentation.			
1. Draws up medication, injects it into piggyback solution This step is not necessary if the medication comes premixed from pharmacy.			
2. Chooses correct tubing and attaches it to the medication bag. Labels the bag with the date, the medication, the dosage, the patient's name, initials, and time given, as needed.			
3. Closes slide clamp on piggyback tubing. Hangs the medication bag on the IV pole.			
4. Squeezes drip chamber, fills it one-third to one-half full.			
5. Opens clamp, primes tubing, holds end of tubing lower than bag of fluid. Does not let more than one drop of fluid escape from end of tubing. Closes clamp.			
"Backflushing" the Piggyback Line:			
a. Alternatively, clamps piggyback tubing, scrubs all surfaces of primary "Y" port, and attaches piggyback setup with needless system.			
b. Opens the clamp on the piggyback tubing and lowers the bag below the primary to prime the piggyback line.			
c. Once line is primed, clamps piggyback tubing.			
6. Labels the tubing with date, medication, dosage, initials of person preparing medication.			
7. Lowers primary IV container to hang below the level of the piggyback IV.			
8. Opens clamp of piggyback line. Regulates drip rate with roller clamp on primary line.			
9. At the end of infusion, clamps piggyback tubing, moves primary tubing back to its original height. Uses roller clamp. Resets primary bag to correct infusion rate.			

Recommendation: Pass _____ Needs more practice _____

Student: _____   Date: _____

Instructor: _____   Date: _____

Check (✔) Yes or No

PROCEDURE STEPS	Yes	No	COMMENTS
Before, during, and after the procedure, follows Principles-Based Checklist to Use With All Procedures, including: Identifies the patient according to agency policy using two identifiers; attends appropriately to standard precautions, hand hygiene, safety, privacy, body mechanics, and documentation.			
1. Obtains the medication. If necessary, draws up medication and injects it into piggyback solution. This step is not necessary if the medication comes premixed from pharmacy.			
2. Hangs the piggyback container on the IV pole. Chooses correct tubing and attaches it to the medication bag, keeping the spike sterile. Labels the bag with the date, the medication, the dosage, and initials, as needed.			
3. Closes slide clamp on piggyback tubing. Squeezes drip chamber, fills it one-third to one-half full.			
4. Opens clamp, primes tubing, holds end of tubing lower than bag of fluid. Does not let more than one drop of fluid escape from end of tubing. Closes clamp.			
Alternatively: "Backflushing" the Piggyback Line:			
a. Connects the medication bag to the primary line.			
b. Pauses the infusion pump. Opens the clamp on the piggyback tubing, lowers the bag below the primary infusion to prime the line, and restarts the pump.			
c. Once the line is primed, clamps the piggyback tubing.			
d. Labels the tubing with date, medication, dosage, initials of person preparing medication.			
e. Hangs piggyback container on IV pole. Lowers primary IV container to hang below the level of the piggyback IV.			
5. Programs the pump by selecting the secondary infusion button. Programs the rate and total volume to be infused.			
6. If backflushing was not used to prime the tubing, scrubs the primary line port, connects the medication line to the primary line, and opens the clamp of the piggyback tubing.			
7. Presses "start" on the infusion pump.			

PROCEDURE STEPS	Yes	No	COMMENTS
8. Checks drip chambers to ensure that the secondary solution is infusing and the primary solution is not.			
9. Checks pump information again to ensure the correct rate and volume.			
10. At the end of infusion, clamps piggyback tubing and checks to see that the pump has changed to the previously programmed primary infusion rate.			

Recommendation: Pass _____ Needs more practice _____

Student: _____   Date: _____

Instructor: _____   Date: _____

PROCEDURE CHECKLIST

Chapter 26: Using a Volume-Control Administration Set (e.g., Buretrol, Volutrol, Soluset)

Check (✔) Yes or No

PROCEDURE STEPS	Yes	No	COMMENTS
Before, during, and after the procedure, follows Principles-Based Checklist to Use With All Procedures, including: Identifies the patient according to agency policy using two identifiers; attends appropriately to standard precautions, hand hygiene, safety, privacy, body mechanics, and documentation.			
1. Prepares volume-control set tubing. a. Closes both upper, lower clamps on tubing.			
b. Opens clamp of the air vent on volume-control chamber.			
c. Maintains sterile procedure, attaches administration spike of volume-control set to primary IV bag.			
d. Fills volume-control chamber with desired amount of IV solution by opening clamp between IV bag and volume-control chamber. When amount of solution is in chamber, closes clamp.			
e. Primes rest of tubing by opening clamp below chamber, running IV fluid until all air has been expelled.			
f. Rechecks amount of fluid in volume control chamber; if needed, adds additional fluid to desired amount.			
2. Vigorously scrubs all surfaces of injection port closest to patient with an antiseptic prep pad.			
3. Connects end of volume-control IV line to patient's IV site. Attaches directly to IV catheter, to extension tubing, or to injection port closest to patient.			
4. Vigorously scrubs injection port on volume-control chamber. Attaches the medication syringe.			
5. Gently rotates chamber to mix medication in IV solution.			
6. Opens lower clamp and starts infusion at correct flow rate.			
7. Labels volume-control chamber with date, time, medication, doses added, initials, according to agency policy.			

PROCEDURE STEPS	Yes	No	COMMENTS
8. When medication has finished infusing, adds a small amount of primary fluid to chamber and flushes tubing. Uses two times volume in dead space of tubing; checks tubing package for amount.			

Recommendation: Pass _____ Needs more practice _____

Student: _____   Date: _____

Instructor: _____   Date: _____

PROCEDURE CHECKLIST
Chapter 27: Administering Feedings Through Gastric and Enteric Tube

Check (✓) Yes or No

PROCEDURE STEPS	Yes	No	COMMENTS
Before, during, and after the procedure, follows Principles-Based Checklist to Use With All Procedures, including: Identifies the patient according to agency policy; attends appropriately to standard precautions, hand hygiene, safety, privacy, and body mechanics.			
1. Checks the health record to determine that tube placement has been confirmed by radiography before the first feeding.			
2. Determines the type of feeding, rate of infusion, and frequency of feeding.			
3. Checks the expiration date of the feeding formula.			
4. Shakes the feeding formula to mix well.			
5. Warms the formula to room temperature for intermittent feedings; for continuous feedings, keeps formula cool but not cold.			
6. Prepares equipment for administration. **For an Open System With Feeding Bag:** a. Fills a disposable tube feeding (TF) bag with a 4- to 6-hour supply of formula; primes the tubing.			
b. Labels the TF bag with date, time, formula type, and rate. Attaches a label "WARNING! For Enteral Use Only—NOT for IV Use." Checks to be sure adapters and connectors used in the enteral system are incompatible with female Luer-Lock rigid connectors used for IV infusion.			
c. Hangs the TF bag on an IV pole.			
For an Open System With Syringe: d. Prepares the syringe by removing the plunger.			
For a Closed System with Prefilled Bottle With Drip Chamber: e. Attaches the administration set to prefilled bottle and primes tubing.			
f. Hangs the prefilled bottle on an IV pole.			
7. Elevates the head of the bed at least 30° to 45°.			

PROCEDURE STEPS	Yes	No	COMMENTS
8. Places a linen saver pad under the connection end of the feeding tube.			
9. Dons procedure gloves.			
10. For the first feeding, after radiography, verifies tube placement by (Clinical Insight, Checking Feeding Tube Placement): a. Aspirating stomach contents and measuring pH.			
b. Asking patient to speak.			
c. Measuring the external length of the tubing.			
d. For nasogastric tubes, but not for gastrostomy or jejunostomy tubes, can additionally confirm by injecting air into the tube and auscultating for "whoosh."			
11. For subsequent feedings, aspirates and measures the gastric residual (except for jejunostomy tubes). a. Connects the syringe to the proximal end of the feeding tube. Draws back slowly to aspirate contents.			
b. Measures the volume of aspirated contents using a syringe (if volume is greater than 60 mL, uses a graduated container).			
c. Reinstills aspirate if there is no abdominal pain or distention.			
d. If the aspirate volume is more than 200 mL, stops the infusion and notifies the primary care provider.			
Variation. Jejunostomy Tubes. Confirms with pH indicator strips and measuring length of tube from naris to connector.			
12. Flushes the feeding tube with 30 mL of tap water (for intermittent feedings).			
Beginning the Feeding:			
13. **If Using an Infusion Pump:** a. Hangs the feeding and prime tubing (unless already done at Step 6). Threads the administration tubing through the infusion pump according to the manufacturer's instructions.			
b. Clamps or pinches off the end of the feeding tube.			
c. If a connector is needed, attaches it to the open end of the feeding tube and connects to the distal end of the administration tubing. If no connector is needed, attaches the distal end of the administration tubing to the proximal (open) end of the feeding tube.			
d. Traces the tubing from the bag back to patient.			
e. Turns on the infusion pump; sets the correct infusion rate and volume to be infused.			

PROCEDURE STEPS	Yes	No	COMMENTS
f. Unclamps the tube and begins infusion.			
14. **If Using an Open System and Syringe:**			
a. Clamps or pinches off the end of the feeding tube.			
b. Attaches the syringe to the proximal (open) end of the feeding tube.			
c. Fills the syringe with the prescribed amount of formula.			
d. Releases the tube clamp or "pinch," and elevates the syringe. Does not elevate syringe greater than 18 inches (45 cm) above the tube insertion site.			
e. Allows feeding to flow slowly (if too fast, lowers the syringe).			
f. When the syringe is nearly empty, clamps the tube or holds it above the level of the stomach; refills the syringe; unclamps and continues feeding until prescribed amount is administered.			
15. **Using a Closed System With a Prefilled Bottle With a Drip Chamber (No Infusion Pump):** a. Pinches or clamps end of feeding tube. b. If connector is needed, attaches to the proximal (open) end of the feeding tube and connects to administration tubing. If no connector is needed, attaches the distal end of the administration tube to the proximal (open) end of the feeding tube. Traces the tubing from the bag back to patient.			
16. Begins the infusion: Opens the roller clamp on the administration tubing and regulates the flow to the prescribed rate (or turns on infusion pump and sets rate and volume to be infused).			
Ending Feeding:			
17. When feeding is infused, proceeds as follows: a. **Infusion Pump** Turns off the pump, pinches the end of the feeding tube, and flushes with the prescribed amount of water.			
b. **Open System Syringe** Disconnects the syringe from the feeding tube, flushes the tube with approximately 50 mL of tap water.			

PROCEDURE STEPS	Yes	No	COMMENTS
c. **Closed System With Prefilled Bottle With Drip Chamber** Turns off the pump or turns the roller clamp off. Disconnects the feeding tube from the administration tubing. Flushes the feeding tube with prescribed amount of water.			
d. **Continuous Feeding** Flushes the tube with the prescribed amount of water (typically 50–100 mL) every 4–6 hours.			
18. Caps the proximal end of the feeding tube.			
19. Keeps the head of the bed elevated at least 30°–45° for 1 hour after TF is infused.			
20. Provides frequent oral hygiene and gargling.			
21. **Procedure Variation for Jejunostomy Tubes:** Does not instill air into the tube nor checks for residual before feeding.			
22. **Procedure Variation for Gastrostomy Tubes and G-Buttons:** Cleans insertion site daily with soap and water. A small, precut, gauze dressing may be applied to site.			
23. **Procedure Variation for Cuffed Tracheostomy Tube:** Inflates the cuff before administering the feeding and keeps the cuff inflated at for least 15 minutes afterward.			

Recommendation: Pass _____ Needs more practice _____

Student: _____   Date: _____

Instructor: _____   Date: _____

 Copyright © 2016, F. A. Davis Company, Wilkinson & Treas/Procedure Checklists for Fundamentals of Nursing, 3e

Check (✓) Yes or No

PROCEDURE STEPS	Yes	No	COMMENTS
Before, during, and after the procedure, follows Principles-Based Checklist to Use With All Procedures, including: Identifies the patient according to agency policy; attends appropriately to standard precautions, hand hygiene, safety, privacy, and body mechanics.			
1. Reviews prescriber's orders, including rate of infusion.			
2. Maintains sterility of tubing and equipment throughout.			
3. Checks patient's blood glucose level before infusing.			
4. Brings equipment and supplies to bedside.			
5. Performs hand hygiene.			
6. Positions patient supine.			
7. Ensures that lipids are not cold.			
8. Examines lipids bottle for leaks, cloudiness, floating particles, brown layer, oil on the surface, or oil droplets. Does not use if present.			
9. Labels the bottle with patient's name, room number, date, time, rate, and start and stop times. Labels the tubing with date and time.			
10. Compares bottle to patient's wrist band (bottle number, expiration date, additives); compares to original prescription. Asks a colleague to verify.			
11. Checks the appearance and patency of the IV insertion site.			
12. Determines patency of the IV line if using a peripheral IV.			
13. Cleanses the stopper on the lipids bottle and allows the surface to dry.			
14. Connects special DEHP-free IV tubing to lipid solution. Uses new tubing for each bottle. (If there is no inline filter, attaches a 1.2-micron filter and extension tubing before priming.)			
15. Primes the tubing.			
16. Places the IV tubing in the infusion pump; sets the pump to the prescribed rate.			

PROCEDURE STEPS	Yes	No	COMMENTS
17. Identifies the correct IV line and port for the infusion. Traces the tubing from the bag back to patient.			
18. Thoroughly scrubs the port site and Luer-Lock threads with an antiseptic pad.			
19. Attaches the infusion tubing to the designated IV port and turns the Luer-Lock to secure the connection.			
20. **Variation:** If a previous bag of lipids is still connected, clamps the catheter lumen and "old" infusion set, quickly disconnects from the venous access device, thoroughly cleanses the port, and connects the new infusion.			
21. Starts the infusion at 1.0 mL/min or as prescribed.			
22. Takes vital signs; repeats every 10 minutes for 30 minutes.			
23. Observes for chills, fever, flushing, dyspnea, nausea, vomiting, headache, and back pain.			
24. Checks again to make sure the catheter–tubing connection is secure.			
25. Takes vital signs. If no reaction occurs, adjusts to the prescribed infusion rate.			
26. Performs hand hygiene.			
27. When the infusion is finished, discards the bottle and the IV administration set.			

Recommendation: Pass _____ Needs more practice _____

Student: _____   Date: _____

Instructor: _____   Date: _____

PROCEDURE CHECKLIST
Chapter 27: Administering Parenteral Nutrition

Check (✓) Yes or No

PROCEDURE STEPS	Yes	No	COMMENTS
Before, during, and after the procedure, follows Principles-Based Checklist to Use With All Procedures, including: Identifies the patient according to agency policy; attends appropriately to standard precautions, hand hygiene, safety, privacy, and body mechanics.			
1. Maintains the sterility of tubing, equipment, and sterile gloves appropriately throughout.			
2. Checks prescriptions for additives and rate of infusion.			
3. Checks patient's blood glucose level (and vital signs if required or needed) before administering.			
4. Checks the appearance and patency of the IV insertion site.			
5. Brings equipment and supplies to the bedside.			
6. Identifies patient, using two identifiers, according to agency policy.			
7. Explains procedure to the patient.			
8. Performs hand hygiene.			
9. Positions patient supine.			
10. Examines PN bag for leaks, cloudiness, and floating particles. If mixed with lipids, examines for brown layer, oil on the surface, or oil droplets. Does not use if present.			
11. Compares bag to patient's wrist band (bag number, expiration date, additives); compares to the original prescription. Asks a colleague to verify.			
12. Connects IV tubing to PN solution. If there is no inline filter, attaches a filter and extension tubing before priming.			
13. Primes the tubing (or primes at Step 14, depending on pump design).			
14. Places the IV tubing in the infusion pump; sets pump to prescribed rate. Primes tubing, if not done at Step 13.			
15. Identifies the correct IV line and lumen for the PN.			
16. Clamps the PN catheter and old PN administration set (if still connected) before disconnecting the tubing.			

PROCEDURE STEPS	Yes	No	COMMENTS
17. Performs hand hygiene.			
18. Dons clean gloves (or sterile, if required by the agency).			
19. Thoroughly scrubs central line injection cap and extension or the Luer-Lock threads on tubing connection, using antiseptic pad (for at least 15–30 seconds).			
20. Determines the patency of the line. Checks for blood return and flushes with saline.			
21. Attaches the infusion tubing to the designated PN port and turns the Luer-Lock to secure the connection.			
22. **Variation:** If a previous infusion is still connected, ensures that the access line is clamped (Step 16), clamps the line to the "old" infusion bag, quickly disconnects it from the central catheter, cleanses the connection, and connects the new bag.			
23. As a final safety check, traces the tubing from the bag back to patient before starting the infusion.			
24. Starts the infusion at the prescribed rate.			
25. Checks again to make sure the catheter–tubing connection is secure.			
26. Labels the tubing with the date and time.			
27. Removes and discards gloves.			
28. Performs hand hygiene.			

Recommendation: Pass _____ Needs more practice _____

Student: _____   Date: _____

Instructor: _____   Date: _____

Check (✓) Yes or No

PROCEDURE STEPS	Yes	No	COMMENTS
Before, during, and after the procedure, follows Principles-Based Checklist to Use With All Procedures, including: Identifies the patient according to agency policy; attends appropriately to standard precautions, hand hygiene, safety, privacy, and body mechanics.			
1. Verifies medical prescription for frequency and timing of testing.			
2. Instructs patient to wash her hands with soap and warm water, if she is able. Lets dry completely.			
3. Turns on the glucose meter. Calibrates according to the manufacturer's instructions.			
4. Checks the expiration date on the container of reagent strips and that it is the correct type for the monitor.			
5. Dons procedure gloves.			
6. Removes the reagent strip from container; tightly seals the container.			
7. Places reagent strip into the glucose meter.			
8. Selects a puncture site on the lateral aspect of a finger (heel or great toe for an infant) and cleans the site with soap and water (or according to facility policy), if the patient was not able to do so. Lets dry completely.			
9. Uses a different site each time glucose is checked.			
10. Positions the finger in a dependent position and massages toward the fingertip.			
11. For infants, older adults, and people with poor circulation, places a warm cloth on the site for about 10 minutes before obtaining the blood sample.			
12. Performs fingerstick:			
a. Engages the sterile injector and removes the cover.			
b. Places a disposable lancet firmly in the end of injector.			
c. Places the back of the hand on the table, or otherwise secures the finger so it does not move when pricked.			
d. Positions the injector firmly against the skin, perpendicular to the puncture site. Pushes the release switch, allowing the needle to pierce the skin.			

PROCEDURE STEPS	Yes	No	COMMENTS
e. If there is no injector, uses a darting motion to prick the site with the lancet.			
13. Lightly squeezes patient's finger above the puncture site until a droplet of blood has collected.			
14. Places a reagent strip test patch close to the drop of blood. Allows contact between the drop of blood and the test patch until blood covers the entire patch. Does not "smear" the blood over the reagent strip.			
15. Inserts the reagent strip into the glucose meter, if not already inserted. (Follows manufacturer's instructions.)			
16. Allows the blood sample to remain in contact with the reagent strip for the amount of time specified by the manufacturer.			
17. Using a gauze pad, gently applies pressure to the puncture site.			
18. After the meter signals, reads the blood glucose level indicated on the digital display.			
19. Turns off the meter and disposes of the reagent strip, cotton ball, gauze pad, paper towel, alcohol pad, and lancet in the proper containers.			
20. Removes the procedure gloves and disposes of them in the proper container.			

Recommendation: Pass _____ Needs more practice _____

Student: _____   Date: _____

Instructor: _____   Date: _____

PROCEDURE CHECKLIST
Chapter 27: Inserting Nasogastric and Nasoenteric Tubes

Check (✓) Yes or No

PROCEDURE STEPS	Yes	No	COMMENTS
Before, during, and after the procedure, follows Principles-Based Checklist to Use With All Procedures, including: Identifies the patient according to agency policy; attends appropriately to standard precautions, hand hygiene, safety, privacy, and body mechanics.			
Pre-Procedure Assessment: Checks patency of nares; chooses appropriate naris.			
1. Prepares the tube. a. Plastic tube: Places in a basin of warm water for 10 minutes (or wraps around index finger).			
b. Rubber tube: Places in a basin of ice for 10 minutes.			
c. Small-bore tube: Inserts stylet or guidewire and secures into position according to agency policy. (Small-bore tubes may come with the guidewire in them.) Leaves the wire in place until tube is positioned and placement checked on x-ray. Once wire is removed, does not reinsert it.			
2. Assists patient into a high Fowler's position, pillow behind head and shoulders. **Variations:** a. If patient is comatose, places patient into a low Fowler's position. Asks a coworker to help position patient's head for insertion.			
b. If patient is confused and combative, asks a coworker to assist with insertion.			
3. Measures the tube length correctly. a. Nasogastric (NG) tube: Measures from the tip of the nose to the earlobe, and from the earlobe to the xiphoid process. Marks the length with tape or indelible ink on the NG tube.			
b. Nasoenteric (NE) tube: Adds 8–10 cm (3–4 in.), or as directed, to NG measurement and marks with tape or indelible ink.			
4. Stands on patient's right side if right-handed and left side if left-handed. Drapes a linen-saver pad over patient's chest and hands him an emesis basin and facial tissues.			
5. Prepares fixation device or cuts a 10-cm (4-in.) piece of hypoallergenic tape; splits the bottom end lengthways.			

PROCEDURE STEPS	Yes	No	COMMENTS
6. Arranges a signal for patient to communicate if he wants to stop.			
7. Dons procedure gloves, if not done previously.			
8. Wraps 10–15 cm (5–6 in.) of end of the tube tightly around index finger, then releases it.			
9. Lubricates the distal 10 cm (4 in.) of the tube with a water-soluble lubricant.			
10. If patient is awake, alert, and able to swallow, hands him a glass of water with a straw.			
11. Instructs patient to hold his head straight up and extend his neck back against the pillow (slight hyperextension).			
12. Begins to insert the NG tube: a. Grasps the tube above the lubricant with the curved end pointing downward.			
b. Gently inserts the tip of the tube along the floor of the nasal passage, on the lateral side, aiming toward the near ear.			
c. If resistance is felt when the tube reaches the nasopharynx, uses gentle pressure, but does not force the tube to advance.			
d. Provides tissues if patient's eyes tear.			
e. Continues insertion until just past the nasopharynx by gently rotating the tube toward the opposite naris.			
13. Pauses briefly for patient to relax; explains that the next step requires him to swallow.			
14. Directs patient to flex his head toward the chest, take a small sip of water, and swallow.			
15. Rotates the tube 180°and directs patient to sip and swallow the water while the nurse slowly advances the tube.			
16. Advances tube 5–10 cm (2–4 in.) with each swallow until marked length is reached. a. If patient gags, stops advancing the tube and instructs patient to take deep breaths and drink a few sips of water.			
b. If gagging continues, uses a tongue blade and penlight to check the tube position in the back of the throat.			
c. If the tube is coiled in the back of the throat, patient coughs excessively during insertion, the tube does not advance with each swallow, or patient develops respiratory distress, withdraws the tube and allows patient to rest before reinserting.			

PROCEDURE STEPS	Yes	No	COMMENTS
d. **Variation: To advance the tube into the small intestine:** After the tube is in the stomach, positions patient on his right side; advances the tube 8–10 cm (3–4 in.) hourly, over several hours (up to 24 hours) until radiography confirms placement.			
17. When the tube is in place, secures it temporarily with one piece of tape so it does not move while the nurse confirms placement.			
18. Verifies tube placement at the bedside by a combination of methods: a. Inspects the posterior pharynx for the presence of coiled tube.			
b. Aspirates stomach contents and measures pH; notes color and consistency of aspirate.			
c. Confirms tube placement by injecting air into the NG tube and auscultating, or asking patient to speak. (Clinical Insight, Checking Feeding Tube Placement)			
d. Asks the patient to speak.			
19. If tube is not in stomach, advances it another 2.5–5 cm (1–2 in.) and repeats Steps 18a through 18d.			
20. After confirming placement, clamps or connects the end of the tube.			
21. Secures the tube with tape or a tube fixation device. *Tape*: a. Applies skin adhesive to patient's nose and allows it to dry.			
b. Using the 5-cm (2-inch) split tape, removes gloves and applies the intact end of the tape to patient's nose.			
c. Wraps the 5-cm (2-in.) strips around the tube where it exits the nose.			
d. Alternatively, uses the 2.5-cm (1-in.) tape; applies one end to patient's nose, wraps the middle around the tube, and secures the other end to the opposite side of the nose.			
Alternative: Uses a fixation device: Places the wide end of the pad over the bridge of the nose; positions the connector around the tube where it exits the nose.			

PROCEDURE STEPS	Yes	No	COMMENTS
22. Curves and tapes the tube to patient's cheek (unless contraindicated by the fixation device).			
23. Ties a slipknot around the tube with a rubber band near the connection; secures the rubber band to patient's gown with a safety pin. Alternatively, uses tape instead of a rubber band.			
24. Elevates the head of the bed to 30° unless contraindicated.			
25. Marks the tube where it enters the naris with tape or indelible ink. Measures the length from the naris to the connector, and records.			

Recommendation: Pass _____ Needs more practice _____

Student: _____   Date: _____

Instructor: _____   Date: _____

PROCEDURE CHECKLIST
Chapter 27: Removing a Nasogastric or Nasoenteric Tube

Check (✓) Yes or No

PROCEDURE STEPS	Yes	No	COMMENTS
Before, during, and after the procedure, follows Principles-Based Checklist to Use With All Procedures, including: Identifies the patient according to agency policy; attends appropriately to standard precautions, hand hygiene, safety, privacy, and body mechanics.			
1. Checks patient's health record to confirm the prescription for removal.			
2. For feeding tubes, waits at least 30 minutes after feeding is finished to remove tube.			
3. Assists patient to a sitting or high Fowler's position.			
4. Places disposable plastic bag on the bed or within reach.			
5. Hands patient facial tissue.			
6. Explains that the procedure may cause some gagging or discomfort, but that it will be brief.			
7. Drapes a linen-saver pad across patient's chest.			
8. Washes hands and dons procedure gloves.			
9. If a nasogastric (NG) tube is connected, turns off suction and disconnects the tube.			
10. Stands on patient's right side if right-handed, and on left side if left-handed.			
11. Attaches the syringe to the proximal end of the NG or NE tube and flushes with 10 mL of air or normal saline.			
12. Unpins the tube from patient's gown and then untapes the tube from patient's nose. Uses adhesive remover as needed.			
13. Clamps or pinches the open end of the tube.			
14. Holds gauze up to patient's nose and is ready to grasp the tube with a towel in the opposite hand. Asks patient to hold his breath.			
15. Quickly, steadily, and smoothly withdraws the tube and places it in the plastic bag.			
16. If patient cannot do so, cleans patient's nares and provides mouth care.			

PROCEDURE STEPS	Yes	No	COMMENTS
17. If the tube was connected to suction, measures the output and notes the characteristics of the content.			
18. Removes gloves and disposes of gloves, tube, and any drainage equipment in the nearest receptacle, according to facility policy.			

Recommendation: Pass _____ Needs more practice _____

Student: _____   Date: _____

Instructor: _____   Date: _____

214   Copyright © 2016, F. A. Davis Company, Wilkinson & Treas/Procedure Checklists for Fundamentals of Nursing, 3e

PROCEDURE CHECKLIST
Chapter 28: Applying a Condom Catheter (Male)

Check (✓) Yes or No

PROCEDURE STEPS	Yes	No	COMMENTS
Before, during, and after the procedure, follows Principles-Based Checklist to Use With All Procedures, including: Identifies patient according to agency policy using two identifiers; attends appropriately to standard precautions, hand hygiene, safety, privacy, and body mechanics.			
1. Dons clean procedure gloves.			
2. Measures the circumference of the penis using a disposable paper tape for correct catheter fit.			
3. Washes hands and dons clean procedure gloves.			
4. Organizes supplies and prepares the bedside drainage bag for attachment to the condom catheter.			
5. Places the patient in a supine position.			
6. Folds down the bedcovers to expose the penis and drapes the patient using the bath blanket.			
7. Gently cleanses the penis with soap and water. Rinses and dries it thoroughly. If the patient is uncircumcised, retracts the foreskin, cleanses the glans, and replaces the foreskin. If the patient has excess hair along the shaft of the penis, carefully clips it with scissors.			
8. Washes hands and changes procedure gloves.			
9. Applies skin prep to the penis and allows it to dry.			
10. Holds the penis in the nondominant hand. With the dominant hand, places the condom catheter at the end of the penis, and slowly unrolls it along the shaft toward the patient's body. Leaves 2.5–5 cm (1–2 in.) between the end of the penis and the drainage tube on the catheter.			
11. Secures the condom catheter in place on the penis, using only the adhesive products supplied with the condom.			
12. Assesses the proximal end of the condom catheter.			
13. Secures the drainage tubing to the patient's thigh using a commercial leg strap or tape.			
14. Covers the patient. Removes gloves and washes hands.			

PROCEDURE STEPS	Yes	No	COMMENTS

Recommendation: Pass _____ Needs more practice _____

Student: _____   Date: _____

Instructor: _____   Date: _____

PROCEDURE CHECKLIST
Chapter 28: Continuous Bladder Irrigation

Check (✓) Yes or No

PROCEDURE STEPS	Yes	No	COMMENTS
Before, during, and after the procedure, follows Principles-Based Checklist to Use With All Procedures, including: Identifies patient according to agency policy using two identifiers; attends appropriately to standard precautions, hand hygiene, safety, privacy, and body mechanics.			
1. Uses sterile irrigation solution, warmed to room temperature.			
2. Never disconnects the drainage tubing from the catheter.			
3. If not already present, inserts a three-way (triple lumen) indwelling catheter.			
4. Prepares the irrigation fluid and tubing: a. Closes the clamp on the connecting tubing.			
b. Spikes the tubing into the appropriate portal on the irrigation solution container, using aseptic technique.			
c. Inverts the container and hangs it on the IV pole.			
d. Removes the protective cap from the distal end of the connecting tubing; holds the end of tubing over a sink and opens the roller clamp slowly, allowing solution to completely fill the tubing. Makes sure to keep the end sterile.			
e. Reclamps the roller on the tubing to stop the flow of the irrigation solution. Recaps the tubing.			
5. Empties urine from the bedside drainage bag and documents the amount.			
6. Performs hand hygiene and dons clean procedure gloves.			
7. Places patient in a supine position and drapes patient so that only the connection port on the indwelling catheter is visible.			
8. Places a waterproof barrier drape under the irrigation port.			

PROCEDURE STEPS	Yes	No	COMMENTS
9. Cleanses the irrigation port with antiseptic swabs. Pinching the tubing and using aseptic technique, connects the end of the irrigation infusion tubing to the irrigation port of the catheter.			
10. Slowly opens the roller clamp on the tubing and regulates the flow of the irrigation solution to meet the desired outcome for the irrigation (e.g., the goal of continuous bladder irrigation for patients who have had a transurethral resection of the prostate is to keep the urine light pink to clear).			
11. Monitors flow rate for 1–2 minutes to ensure accuracy.			
12. Removes gloves; washes hands.			
13. Assists the patient to a comfortable position.			

Recommendation: Pass _____ Needs more practice _____

Student: _____   Date: _____

Instructor: _____   Date: _____

PROCEDURE CHECKLIST
Chapter 28: Inserting an Indwelling Urinary Catheter (Female)

Check (✓) Yes or No

PROCEDURE STEPS	Yes	No	COMMENTS
Before, during, and after the procedure, follows Principles-Based Checklist to Use With All Procedures, including: Identifies patient according to agency policy using two identifiers; attends appropriately to standard precautions, hand hygiene, safety, privacy, and body mechanics.			
1. Takes an extra pair of sterile gloves and an extra sterile catheter into the room.			
2. Ensures good lighting.			
3. Works on the right side of the bed if right-handed; the left side if left-handed.			
4. Places patient in a dorsal recumbent position (supine). a. Asks her to flex her knees and place her feet flat on the bed. b. Instructs the patient to relax her thighs and allow them to rotate externally.			
5. If patient is confused or unable to follow directions, obtains help.			
6. Drapes patient. Covers upper body with blanket. Folds the blanket in a diamond shape, wrapping the corners around the patient's legs and folding the upper corner down over the perineum.			
7. Lifts the corner of the privacy drape to expose the perineum.			
8. Positions the procedure light to allow optimal visualization of the perineum and then locates the urinary meatus.			
9. Dons procedure gloves. Washes the perineal area with soap and water. Lets it dry.			
10. Removes and discards gloves.			
11. Washes hands.			
12. Organizes the work area: a. Bedside or overbed table within nurse's reach.			
b. Opens the sterile catheter kit and places on the bedside or overbed table, without contaminating the inside of the wrap.			

PROCEDURE STEPS	Yes	No	COMMENTS
c. Positions a plastic bag or other trash receptacle so that nurse does not have to reach across the sterile field (e.g., near the patient's feet); or places a trash can on the floor beside the bed.			
13. Applies a sterile underpad and drape. *Variation*: Sterile underpad packed as top item in the kit			
a. Removes the sterile underpad from the kit before donning sterile gloves. Does not touch other kit items with bare hands.			
b. Allows the drape to fall open as it is removed from the kit. Touching only the corners, places the drape shiny side down under the patient's buttocks.			
c. Carefully removes the sterile glove package from the kit and dons sterile gloves.			
d. Picks up the fenestrated drape; allows it to unfold without touching other objects; places over the perineum with the hole over the labia. (The fenestrated drape is considered optional in some facilities.)			
Variation: Sterile gloves packed as top item in the kit			
Uses the following steps instead of Steps 13a–d: e. Removes the sterile glove package from the kit and dons sterile gloves. f. Grasps the edges of the sterile underpad. Folds the entire edge down 5–7.5 cm (2–3 in.), making a cuff to protect the gloves. Asks the patient to raise her hips slightly if she is able. Carefully slides the drape under the patient's buttocks without contaminating the gloves. g. Picks up the fenestrated drape; allows it to unfold without touching other objects; places over the perineum with the hole over the labia. (The fenestrated drape is considered optional in some facilities.)			
14. Organizes kit supplies on the sterile field and prepares the supplies in the kit, maintaining sterility. a. Opens the antiseptic packet; pours solution over the cotton balls. (Some kits contain sterile antiseptic swabs; if so, opens the "stick" end of the packet.)			

b. Lays forceps near cotton balls (omits step if using swabs).			
c. Opens the specimen container if a specimen is to be collected.			
d. Removes any unneeded supplies (e.g., specimen container) from the field.			
e. Removes the plastic wrapper from the catheter, if it is covered.			
f. Squeezes the sterile lubricant into the kit tray. Rolls the catheter slowly in the lubricant, being sure to generously lubricate the first 2.5–5 cm (1–2 in.) of the catheter. Leaves the catheter tip in the sterile lubricant or on the sterile field until ready to use.			
g. Attaches the sterile water-filled syringe to the balloon port of the catheter. Leaves the syringe attached to the catheter.			
15. Touching only the kit or inside of the wrapping, places the sterile catheter kit down onto the sterile field between the patient's legs.			
16. If the drainage bag is preconnected to the catheter, leaves the bag on the sterile field until after the catheter is inserted.			
17. Places the nondominant hand above the labia, and, with thumb and forefinger, spreads the patient's labia, pulling up at the same time to expose the urinary meatus. Uses firm pressure to hold this position throughout the procedure.			
18. If the labia accidentally slip back over the meatus during cleansing, repeats the procedure.			
19. Continuing to spread the labia with the nondominant hand, holds forceps in the dominant hand and picks up a cotton ball.			
20. Wipes from the clitoris to the anus, wiping in the order of: far labium majora, near labium majora, inside far labium, inside near labium, and directly down the center over the urinary meatus. Uses only one stroke and a new cotton ball or swab for each area. *Note*: If the kit has only three cotton balls, cleanses only the inside far labium minora, the inside near labium minora, and down the center of the urethral meatus.			

21. Discards cotton balls or swabs as they are used; does not move them across the open sterile kit and field.			
22. With the dominant hand, holds the catheter 5–7.5 cm (2–3 in.) from the tip, with the remainder of the catheter coiled in the palm of the hand.			
23. Asks patient to bear down as though trying to void; slowly inserts the end of the catheter into the meatus. Asks the patient to take slow, deep breaths until the initial discomfort has passed.			
24. Continues gentle insertion of catheter until urine flows. This is about 5–7.5 cm (2–3 in.) in a woman. Then inserts the catheter another 2.5–5 cm (1–2 in.).			
25. If resistance is felt, withdraws the catheter; does not force the catheter.			
26. After urine flows, stabilizes the catheter's position in the urethra with nondominant hand; uses the dominant hand to pick up sterile water-filled syringe and inflates the catheter balloon.			
27. If patient complains of severe pain upon inflation of the balloon, the balloon is probably in the urethra. Allows the water to drain out of the balloon, and advances the catheter 2.5 cm (1 in.) farther into the bladder. After the balloon is inflated, pulls back gently on the catheter until resistance is felt.			
28. If it is not preconnected, connects the drainage bag to the end of the catheter.			
29. Hangs the drainage bag on the side of the bed below the level of the bladder.			
30. Using a commercial catheter securement device (such as a cath tube holder or Velcro leg strap) or hypoallergenic tape, secures the catheter to the thigh.			
31. Cleanses patient's perineal area as needed, and dries.			
32. Discards supplies in a biohazard receptacle.			
33. Removes gloves; washes hands.			
34. Returns patient to a position of comfort.			

Recommendation: Pass _____ Needs more practice _____

Student: _____   Date: _____

Instructor: _____   Date: _____

222   Copyright © 2016, F. A. Davis Company, Wilkinson & Treas/Procedure Checklists for Fundamentals of Nursing, 3e

PROCEDURE CHECKLIST
Chapter 28: Inserting an Indwelling Urinary Catheter (Male)

Check (✓) Yes or No

PROCEDURE STEPS	Yes	No	COMMENTS
Before, during, and after the procedure, follows Principles-Based Checklist to Use With All Procedures, including: Identifies patient according to agency policy using two identifiers; attends appropriately to standard precautions, hand hygiene, safety, privacy, and body mechanics.			
1. Takes an extra pair of sterile gloves and an extra sterile catheter into the room.			
2. Works on the right side of the bed if right-handed and on the left side if left-handed.			
3. Places patient supine, legs straight and slightly apart.			
4. If patient is confused or unable to follow directions, obtains help.			
5. Drapes patient. Covers upper body with blanket; folds linens down to expose the penis.			
6. Dons clean procedure gloves and washes the penis and perineal area with soap and water.			
7. If using topical anesthetic gel for the procedure, uses a needleless syringe and inserts it into the urethra.			
8. Removes and discards gloves.			
9. Washes hands.			
10. Organizes the work area: a. Bedside or overbed table within nurse's reach.			
b. Opens the sterile catheter kit and places on the bedside or overbed table, without contaminating the inside of the wrap.			
c. Positions a plastic bag or other trash receptacle so that nurse does not have to reach across the sterile field (e.g., near the patient's feet); or places a trash can on the floor beside the bed.			
11. Applies sterile underpad and drape. *Variation*: Sterile underpad packed as the top item in the kit			
a. Removes the sterile underpad from the kit before donning sterile gloves. Does not touch other kit items with bare hands.			

PROCEDURE STEPS	Yes	No	COMMENTS
b. Allows the drape to fall open as it is removed from the kit. Touching only the corners, places the drape shiny side down across the patient's thighs.			
c. Carefully removes the sterile glove package from the kit and dons sterile gloves.			
d. Picks up the fenestrated drape; allows it to unfold without touching other objects; places the hole over the penis.			
Variation: Sterile gloves packed as top item in the kit			
Uses the following steps instead of Steps 11a–d: e. Removes the sterile glove package from the kit and dons sterile gloves. f. Grasps the edges of the sterile underpad and carefully places it shiny side down across the patient's thighs. g. Picks up the fenestrated drape; allows it to unfold without touching other objects; places the center hole over the penis.			
12. Organizes kit supplies on the sterile field and prepares the supplies in the kit, maintaining sterility. a. Opens the antiseptic packet; pours solution over the cotton balls. (Some kits contain sterile antiseptic swabs; if so, opens the "stick" end of the packet.)			
b. Lays forceps near cotton balls (omits step if using swabs).			
c. Opens the specimen container if a specimen is to be collected.			
d. Removes any unneeded supplies (e.g., specimen container) from the field.			
e. Removes the plastic wrapper from the catheter, if it is covered.			
f. If the lubricant comes in a packet, squeezes the lubricant into the kit tray and rolls the catheter slowly in the lubricant. Generously lubricates the first 12.5–17.5 cm (5–7 in.) of the catheter. Leaves the catheter tip in sterile lubricant or on the sterile field until ready to use. Does not lubricate the catheter if topical anesthetic gel has already been inserted into the urethra, or if lubricant will be inserted via syringe into the urethra.			

PROCEDURE STEPS	Yes	No	COMMENTS
g. Attaches the sterile water-filled syringe to the balloon port of the catheter. Leaves the syringe attached to the catheter.			
13. Touching only the kit or inside of the wrapping, places the sterile catheter kit down onto the sterile field between or on top of the patient's thighs.			
14. If the drainage bag is preconnected to the catheter, leaves the bag on the sterile field until after the catheter is inserted.			
15. With the nondominant hand, reaches through the opening in the fenestrated drape and grasps the penis, taking care not to contaminate the surrounding drape. If the penis is uncircumcised, retracts foreskin to expose the meatus. Holds the penis gently, but firmly, at a 90° angle to the body exerting gentle traction.			
16. If the foreskin accidentally falls back over the meatus, or if the nurse drops the penis during cleansing, repeats the procedure.			
17. Continuing to hold the penis with the nondominant hand, holds forceps in the dominant hand and picks up a cotton ball.			
18. Cleanses the glans in a series of circular motions, starting at the meatus and working partially down the shaft of the penis.			
19. Repeats with at least two more cotton balls or swabs.			
20. Discards cotton balls or swabs as they are used; does not move them across the open, sterile kit and field.			
21. Lubrication (if not done previously with a topical anesthetic gel). *Variation:* Lubricant packaged in a syringe Gently inserts the tip of the prefilled syringe into the urethra and instills the lubricant. *Variation:* Lubricant in a packet Checks that the catheter has been generously lubricated for a distance of 12.5–17.5 cm (5– 7 in.).			
22. With the dominant hand, holds the catheter 5–7.5 cm (2–3 in.) from the tip with the remainder of the catheter coiled in the palm of the hand.			

PROCEDURE STEPS	Yes	No	COMMENTS
23. Continues to hold the penis gently but firmly at a 90° angle to the body with the nondominant hand, exerting gentle traction. Asks patient to bear down as though trying to void; slowly inserts the end of the catheter into the meatus. Instructs patient to take slow, deep breaths until the initial discomfort has passed.			
24. Continues gentle insertion of the catheter until urine flows. This is about 17.5–22.5 cm (7–9 in.) in a man. Continues to advance almost to the bifurcation (Y connector).			
25. If resistance is felt at the prostatic sphincter, holds the catheter firmly against the sphincter until it relaxes. Then advances catheter, but does not force it.			
26. After urine flows, stabilizes the catheter's position in the urethra with the nondominant hand; uses the dominant hand to pick up sterile water–filled syringe and inflates the catheter balloon.			
27. If patient complains of pain upon inflation of the balloon, the balloon is probably in the urethra. Allows the water to drain out of the balloon, and advances the catheter 2.5 cm (1 in.) farther into the bladder. After the balloon is inflated, pulls back gently on the catheter until resistance is felt.			
28. If it is not preconnected, connects the drainage bag to the end of the catheter.			
29. Hangs the drainage bag on the side of the bed below the level of the bladder.			
30. Using a commercial catheter securement device (such as a catheter tube holder or Velcro leg strap) or hypoallergenic tape, secures the catheter to the thigh or the abdomen.			
31. Cleanses patient's penis and perineal area as needed, and dries. Replaces foreskin over end of penis.			
32. Discards supplies in an appropriate receptacle.			
33. Removes gloves; washes hands.			
34. Returns patient to a position of comfort.			

Recommendation: Pass _____ Needs more practice _____

Student: _____   Date: _____

Instructor: _____   Date: _____

PROCEDURE CHECKLIST
Chapter 28: Inserting an Intermittent (Straight) Urinary Catheter (Male)

Check (✓) Yes or No

PROCEDURE STEPS	Yes	No	COMMENTS
Before, during, and after the procedure, follows Principles-Based Checklist to Use With All Procedures, including: Identifies patient according to agency policy using two identifiers; attends appropriately to standard precautions, hand hygiene, safety, privacy, and body mechanics.			
1. Takes an extra pair of sterile gloves and an extra sterile catheter into the room.			
2. Works on the right side of the bed if right-handed and on the left side if left-handed.			
3. Places patient supine, legs straight and slightly apart.			
4. If patient is confused or unable to follow directions, obtains help.			
5. Drapes patient. Covers upper body with blanket; folds linens down to expose the penis.			
6. Dons clean procedure gloves and washes the penis and perineal area with soap and water.			
7. If using a topical anesthetic gel for the procedure, uses a needleless syringe and inserts it into the urethra.			
8. Removes and discards gloves.			
9. Washes hands.			
10. Organizes the work area: a. Bedside or overbed table within nurse's reach.			
b. Opens the sterile catheter kit and places on the bedside or overbed table without contaminating the inside of the wrap.			
c. Positions a plastic bag or other trash receptacle so that nurse does not have to reach across the sterile field (e.g., near patient's feet); or places a trash can on the floor beside the bed.			
11. Applies sterile underpad and drape. *Variation*: Sterile underpad packed as top item in the kit			
a. Removes the sterile underpad from the kit before donning sterile gloves. Does not touch other kit items with bare hands.			

PROCEDURE STEPS	Yes	No	COMMENTS
b. Allows the drape to fall open as it is removed from the kit. Touching only the corners, places the drape shiny side down across the patient's thighs.			
c. Carefully removes the sterile glove package from the kit and dons sterile gloves.			
d. Picks up the fenestrated drape; allows it to unfold without touching other objects; places the hole over the penis.			
Variation: Sterile gloves packed as top item in the kit. Uses the following steps instead of Steps 11a–d:			
e. Removes the sterile glove package from the kit and dons sterile gloves.			
f. Grasps the edges of the sterile underpad and carefully places it shiny side down across the patient's thighs.			
g. Picks up the fenestrated drape; allows it to unfold without touching other objects; places the center hole over the penis.			
h. Places the fenestrated drape so that the hole is over the penis.			
12. Organizes kit supplies on the sterile field and prepares the supplies in the kit, maintaining sterility. a. Opens the antiseptic packet; pours solution over the cotton balls. (Some kits contain sterile antiseptic swabs; if so, opens the "stick" end of the packet.)			
b. Lays forceps near cotton balls (omits step if kit includes swabs).			
c. Opens the specimen container if a specimen is to be collected.			
d. Removes any unneeded supplies (e.g., specimen container) from the field.			
e. Removes the plastic wrapper from the catheter, if it is covered.			

PROCEDURE STEPS	Yes	No	COMMENTS
f. If the lubricant comes in a packet, squeezes the lubricant into the kit tray and rolls the catheter slowly in the lubricant. Generously lubricates the first 12.5–17.5 cm (5–7 in.) of the catheter. Leaves the catheter tip in sterile lubricant or on the sterile field until ready to use. *Variation:* Lubricant packaged in a syringe Gently inserts the tip of the prefilled syringe into the urethra and instills the lubricant. *Variation:* Lubricant in a packet Does not lubricate the catheter if a topical anesthetic gel has already been inserted into the urethra or if lubricant will be inserted via syringe into the urethra.			
13. Touching only the kit or inside of the wrapping, places the sterile catheter kit down onto the sterile field between or on top of the patient's thighs.			
14. With the nondominant hand, reaches through the opening in the fenestrated drape and grasps the penis, taking care not to contaminate the surrounding drape. If the penis is uncircumcised, retracts foreskin to expose the meatus. Holds the penis gently, but firmly, at a 90° angle to the body exerting gentle traction.			
15. If the foreskin accidentally falls back over the meatus, or if the nurse drops the penis during cleansing, repeats the procedure.			
16. Continuing to hold the penis with the nondominant hand, holds forceps in dominant hand and picks up a cotton ball.			
17. Cleanses the glans in a series of circular motions, starting at the meatus and working partially down the shaft of the penis.			
18. Repeats with at least two more cotton balls or swabs.			
19. Discards cotton balls or swabs as they are used; does not move them across the open, sterile kit and field.			
20. Maintaining sterile technique, places the plastic urine receptacle close enough to the urinary meatus for the end of the catheter to rest inside the container as the urine drains (e.g., places container between patient's thighs).			
21. With the dominant hand, holds the catheter 5–7.5 cm (2–3 in.) from the tip with remainder coiled in the palm of the hand. Ensures that the distal end of the catheter is in the plastic container.			

PROCEDURE STEPS	Yes	No	COMMENTS
22. Continues to hold the penis gently but firmly at a 90° angle to the body with the nondominant hand, exerting gentle traction. Asks the patient to bear down as though trying to void; slowly inserts the end of the catheter into the meatus. Instructs the patient to take slow, deep breaths until the initial discomfort has passed.			
23. Continues gentle insertion of catheter until urine flows. This is about 17.5–22.5 cm (7–9 in.) in a man. Then inserts the catheter another 2.5–5 cm (1–2 in.).			
24. If resistance is felt at the prostatic sphincter, holds the catheter firmly against the sphincter until it relaxes. Then advances the catheter, but does not force it.			
25. Continues to hold the penis and catheter securely with the nondominant hand while the urine drains from the bladder.			
26. If a urine specimen is to be collected, uses the dominant hand to place the specimen container into the flow of urine; caps container using sterile technique.			
27. When the flow of urine has ceased and the bladder has been emptied, pinches the catheter and slowly withdraws it from the meatus.			
28. Removes the urine-filled receptacle and sets aside to be measured and emptied when the procedure is finished.			
29. Cleanses and dries patient's penis and perineal area as needed; replaces foreskin over end of penis.			
30. Discards supplies in an appropriate receptacle.			
31. Removes gloves; washes hands.			
32. Returns patient to a position of comfort.			

Recommendation: Pass _____ Needs more practice _____

Student: _____   Date: _____

Instructor: _____   Date: _____

PROCEDURE CHECKLIST
Chapter 28: Inserting an Intermittent (Straight) Urinary Catheter (Female)

Check (✓) Yes or No

PROCEDURE STEPS	Yes	No	COMMENTS
Before, during, and after the procedure, follows Principles-Based Checklist to Use With All Procedures, including: Identifies patient according to agency policy using two identifiers; attends appropriately to standard precautions, hand hygiene, safety, privacy, and body mechanics.			
1. Takes an extra pair of sterile gloves and an extra sterile catheter into the room.			
2. Ensures good lighting.			
3. Works on the right side of the bed if right-handed and on the left side if left-handed.			
4. Places the patient in a dorsal recumbent position (supine). 　a. Asks her to flex her knees and place her feet flat on the bed. 　b. Instructs the patient to relax her thighs and allow them to rotate externally.			
5. If patient is confused or unable to follow directions, obtains help.			
6. Dons clean procedure gloves. Drapes patient. Covers upper body with blanket. Folds the blanket in a diamond shape, wrapping the corners around the patient's legs and folding the upper corner down over the perineum.			
7. Lifts the corner of the privacy drape to expose the perineum.			
8. Positions the procedure light to allow optimal visualization of the perineum and then locates the urinary meatus.			
9. Washes the perineal area with perineal wash solution. Lets it dry.			
10. Removes and discards gloves.			
11. Washes hands.			
12. Organizes the work area: 　a. Bedside or overbed table within nurse's reach.			
b. Opens the sterile catheter kit and places on the bedside or overbed table without contaminating the inside of the wrap.			

PROCEDURE STEPS	Yes	No	COMMENTS
c. Positions a plastic bag or other trash receptacle so that nurse does not have to reach across the sterile field (e.g., near the patient's feet); or places a trash can on the floor beside the bed.			
13. Applies a sterile underpad and drape. *Variation*: Sterile underpad packed as top item in the kit			
a. Removes the sterile underpad from the kit before donning sterile gloves. Does not touch other kit items with bare hands.			
b. Allows the drape to fall open as it is removed from the kit. Touching only the corners, places the drape shiny side down under the patient's buttocks.			
c. Carefully removes the sterile glove package from the kit and dons sterile gloves.			
d. Picks up the fenestrated drape; allows it to unfold without touching other objects; places over the perineum with the hole over the labia. (The fenestrated drape is considered optional in some facilities.)			
Variation: Sterile gloves packed as top item in the kit. Uses the following steps instead of Steps 13a–d:			
e. Removes the sterile glove package from the kit and dons sterile gloves.			
f. Grasps the edges of the sterile underpad. Folds the entire edge down 5–7.5 cm (2–3 in.), making a cuff to protect the gloves. Asks the patient to raise her hips slightly if she is able. Carefully slides the drape under the patient's buttocks without contaminating the gloves.			
g. Picks up the fenestrated drape; allows it to unfold without touching other objects; places over the perineum with the hole over the labia. (The fenestrated drape is considered optional in some facilities.)			
14. Organizes kit supplies on the sterile field and prepares the supplies in the kit, maintaining sterility. a. Opens the antiseptic packet; pours solution over the cotton balls. (Some kits contain sterile antiseptic swabs; if so, opens the "stick" end of the packet.)			

PROCEDURE STEPS	Yes	No	COMMENTS
b. Lays forceps near cotton balls (omits step if using swabs).			
c. Opens the specimen container if a specimen is to be collected.			
d. Removes any unneeded supplies (e.g., specimen container) from the field.			
e. Removes the plastic wrapper from the catheter, if it is covered.			
f. Squeezes the sterile lubricant into the kit tray. Rolls the catheter slowly in the lubricant, being sure to generously lubricate the first 2.5–5 cm (1–2 in.) of the catheter. Leaves the catheter tip in the sterile lubricant or on the sterile field until ready to use.			
15. Touching only the kit or the inside of the wrapping, places the sterile catheter kit down onto the sterile field between patient's legs.			
16. Places the nondominant hand above the labia and, with thumb and forefinger, spreads the patient's labia, pulling up at the same time to expose the urinary meatus. Uses firm pressure to hold this position throughout the procedure.			
17. If the labia accidentally slip back over the meatus during cleansing, repeats the procedure.			
18. Continuing to spread the labia with the nondominant hand, holds forceps in the dominant hand and picks up a cotton ball.			
19. Wipes from the clitoris to the anus, wiping in the order of: far labium majora, near labium majora, inside far labium, inside near labium, and directly down the center over the urinary meatus. Uses only one stroke and a new cotton ball or swab for each area. *Note*: If the kit has only three cotton balls, cleanses only the inside far labium minora, the inside near labium minora, and down the center of the urethral meatus.			
20. Discards cotton balls or swabs as they are used; does not move them across the open, sterile kit and field.			
21. Maintaining sterile technique, places the urine receptacle close enough to the urinary meatus, about 10 cm (4 in.) away, for the end of the catheter to rest inside the container as the urine drains.			

PROCEDURE STEPS	Yes	No	COMMENTS
22. With the dominant hand, holds the catheter 5–7.5 cm (2– 3 in.) from the tip, with the remainder of the catheter coiled in the palm of the hand. Ensures that the distal end of the catheter is in the plastic container.			
23. Asks patient to bear down as though trying to void; slowly inserts the end of the catheter into the meatus. Asks the patient to take slow, deep breaths until the initial discomfort has passed.			
24. Continues gentle insertion of catheter until urine flows. This is about 5–7.5 cm (2–3 in.) in a woman. Then inserts the catheter another 2.5–5 cm (1–2 in.).			
25. If resistance is felt, withdraws the catheter; does not force the catheter.			
26. Continues to hold the catheter securely with the nondominant hand while urine drains from the bladder.			
27. If a urine specimen is to be collected, uses the dominant hand to place the specimen container into the flow of urine; caps container using sterile technique.			
28. When the flow of urine has ceased and the bladder has been emptied, pinches the catheter and slowly withdraws it from the meatus.			
29. Removes the urine-filled receptacle and sets aside to be measured and emptied when the procedure is finished.			
30. Cleanses and dries the patient's perineal area as needed.			
31. Discards supplies in an appropriate receptacle.			
32. Removes gloves; washes hands.			
33. Returns patient to a position of comfort.			

Recommendation: Pass _____ Needs more practice _____

Student: _____   Date: _____

Instructor: _____   Date: _____

PROCEDURE CHECKLIST
Chapter 28: Intermittent Bladder Irrigation

Check (✓) Yes or No

PROCEDURE STEPS	Yes	No	COMMENTS
Before, during, and after the procedure, follows Principles-Based Checklist to Use With All Procedures, including: Identifies patient according to agency policy using two identifiers; attends appropriately to standard precautions, hand hygiene, safety, privacy, and body mechanics.			
1. Uses sterile irrigation solution, warmed to room temperature.			
2. Never disconnects the drainage tubing from the catheter.			
Intermittent Irrigation, Three-Way (Triple-Lumen) Indwelling Catheter			
3. If not already present, inserts a three-way (triple lumen) indwelling catheter.			
4. Prepares the irrigation fluid and tubing: a. Closes the clamp on the connecting tubing.			
b. Spikes the tubing into the appropriate portal on the irrigation solution container, using aseptic technique.			
c. Inverts the container and hangs it on the IV pole.			
d. Removes the protective cap from the distal end of the connecting tubing; holds end of tubing over a sink and opens the roller clamp slowly, allowing solution to completely fill the tubing. Makes sure to keep the end sterile.			
e. Reclamps the roller on the tubing to stop the flow of the irrigation solution. Recaps the tubing.			
5. Empties urine from the bedside drainage bag and documents the amount.			
6. Performs hand hygiene and dons clean procedure gloves.			
7. Places patient in a supine position and drapes patient so that only the connection port on the indwelling catheter is visible.			

PROCEDURE STEPS	Yes	No	COMMENTS
8. Places a waterproof barrier drape under the irrigation port.			
9. Scrubs the irrigation port with antiseptic swabs. Pinching the tubing and using aseptic technique, connects the end of the irrigation infusion tubing to the irrigation port of the catheter.			
10. Slowly opens the roller clamp on the irrigation tubing to the desired flow rate.			
11. Instills or irrigates with the prescribed amount of irrigant. If the irrigant is to remain in the bladder for a certain time period, clamps the drainage tubing for that time.			
12. When the correct amount of irrigant has been used and/or the goals of the irrigation have been met, closes the roller clamp on the irrigation tubing, leaving the tubing connected to the catheter for use during the next irrigation.			
13. Removes gloves; washes hands.			
14. Returns patient to a comfortable position.			
Intermittent Irrigation, Two-Way Indwelling Catheter			
15. Follows Steps 1–2, above.			
16. Dons clean procedure gloves; empties any urine currently in the bedside drainage bag.			
17. Washes hands and applies clean gloves.			
18. Places patient in a supine position and drapes patient so that only the specimen removal port on the drainage tubing is exposed.			
19. Places a waterproof drape beneath the exposed port.			
20. Opens the sterile irrigation supplies. Pours approximately 100 mL of the irrigating solution into the sterile container, using aseptic technique.			
21. Draws irrigation solution into the syringe. (For catheter irrigation, uses a total of 15–20 mL; for bladder irrigation the amount is usually 30–60 mL.)			
22. Scrubs all surfaces of the specimen removal port with an antiseptic swab.			

PROCEDURE STEPS	Yes	No	COMMENTS
23. Clamps or pinches the drainage tubing distal to the specimen port.			
24. Inserts the needleless access device into the specimen port and injects the solution, holding the specimen port slightly above the level of the bladder.			
25. If resistance is met, asks patient to turn slightly and attempts a second time. If resistance continues, stops the procedure and notifies the physician.			
26. When the irrigant has been injected, removes the syringe. Refills the syringe if necessary.			
27. Repeats the irrigation until the prescribed amount is instilled.			
28. Unclamps the drainage tubing and allows the irrigant and urine to flow into the bedside drainage bag by gravity. (If the solution is to remain in the bladder for a prescribed time, leaves the tubing clamped for that time period.)			
29. Removes gloves; washes hands.			
30. Returns patient to a position of comfort.			

Recommendation: Pass _____ Needs more practice _____

Student: _____ Date: _____

Instructor: _____ Date: _____

PROCEDURE CHECKLIST
Chapter 28: Measuring Urine

Check (✓) Yes or No

PROCEDURE STEPS	Yes	No	COMMENTS
Before, during, and after the procedure, follows Principles-Based Checklist to Use With All Procedures, including: Identifies patient according to agency policy using two identifiers; attends appropriately to standard precautions, hand hygiene, safety, privacy, and body mechanics.			
Measuring Urine Output From a Bedpan or Urinal			
1. Washes hands and dons clean procedure gloves.			
2. Places a bedpan or urinal in the appropriate position as indicated.			
3. Removes the bedpan or urinal, being careful not to spill the urine. Repositions patient and transports the urine to the bathroom.			
4. While wearing clean gloves, pours the urine into a graduated cylinder or calibrated measuring container, labeled with the correct patient information (in many institutions, labels are preprinted or bar-coded).			
5. Places the measuring device on a flat surface (e.g., shelf, table) and reads the amount at eye level.			
6. Discards the urine in the toilet. If a specimen is required, transfers 30–60 mL of urine to the designated container.			
7. Cleans the measuring container and stores in the patient's bathroom.			
8. Removes gloves and washes hands.			
9. Records the time and volume on the I&O record, and records observations of urine color, clarity, and odor.			
Measuring Urine From an Indwelling Catheter			
1. While wearing clean gloves, places the drainage spout for the collection bag inside a calibrated measuring device. Avoids touching the spout to the inside of the container.			
2. Unclamps the drainage spout and directs the flow of urine into the measuring device.			
3. Reclamps the spout when the collection bag is empty.			
4. Wipes the drainage spout with an alcohol pad and replaces the spout into the slot on the collection bag.			

PROCEDURE STEPS	Yes	No	COMMENTS
5. Measures urine output from the indwelling catheter at the end of each shift unless otherwise ordered.			
6. Discards the urine in the toilet.			
7. Removes gloves and washes hands.			
8. Records the time and amount on the I&O record; records observations of urine color, clarity, and odor.			
Measuring Post-Void Residual Urine Volume Utilizing a Portable Bladder Scanner			
1. Performs hand hygiene and applies clean gloves.			
2. Assists the patient to a supine position. Uncovers only the patient's lower abdomen and suprapubic area.			
3. Cleans the scanner head with antiseptic wipes.			
4. Turns the device on.			
5. Selects the patient's gender. If a woman has had a hysterectomy, follows the manufacturer's directions for gender selection.			
6. Palpates the symphysis pubis and applies ultrasound gel midline on the abdomen, approximately 2.5–4 cm (1–1.5 in.) above the symphysis pubis.			
7. Positions the scanner head in the gel and aims it towards the bladder, pointing slightly downward toward the patient's coccyx.			
8. Presses and releases the "SCAN" button. Holds the scanner head steady until the scan is finished.			
9. Reads the bladder volume measurement. Repeats the scan several times to ensure accuracy. If the scanner shows an image of the bladder, makes sure that the image is centered on the crossbars. If it is not, repositions the scanner head and repeats the scan.			
10. Presses "DONE" when finished. Prints the results by pressing "PRINT."			
11. Wipes the gel from the patient's skin; covers the patient and returns to a comfortable position.			
12. Cleans the scanner head with an antiseptic wipe.			
13. Removes gloves and performs hand hygiene.			

Recommendation: Pass _____ Needs more practice _____

Student: _____ Date: _____

Instructor: _____ Date: _____

PROCEDURE CHECKLIST
Chapter 28: Obtaining a Clean Catch Urine Specimen

Check (✓) Yes or No

PROCEDURE STEPS	Yes	No	COMMENTS
Before, during, and after the procedure, follows Principles-Based Checklist to Use With All Procedures, including: Identifies patient according to agency policy using two identifiers; attends appropriately to standard precautions, hand hygiene, safety, privacy, and body mechanics.			
Note: If patient can do self-care, instructs patient in the following steps. If not, performs them for the patient.			
1. Washes hands and dons clean procedure gloves.			
2. Washes the perineal area with warm water and mild soap, if soiled. Allows the area to dry.			
3. Removes soiled gloves, washes hands, and dons clean procedure gloves.			
4. Opens the prepackaged kit (if available) and removes the contents. Opens the sterile specimen cup, being careful not to touch the inside of the lid or container, and places within easy reach. Makes sure to place the lid with the inside surface facing upward.			
Variation: For Women			
a. Opens the antiseptic towelettes provided in the prepackaged kit. If there is no kit, pours the antiseptic solution over the cotton balls. Spreads the labia and wipes down one side of the meatus from front to back using one pad and discards it. Then wipes the other side with a second pad. Wipes down the center over the urinary meatus with the third pad; then discards it. Maintains separation of the labia until the specimen is obtained.			
Variation: For Men			
b. If the penis is uncircumcised, retracts the foreskin back from the end of the penis.			
c. Uses the towelettes provided in the prepackaged kit or pours antiseptic solution over cotton balls or 2 in.×2 in. gauze pads.			

PROCEDURE STEPS	Yes	No	COMMENTS
d. With one hand, grasps the penis gently. With the other hand, cleanses the meatus in a circular motion from the meatus outward, and cleanses for a few inches down the shaft of the penis. Repeats this cleaning procedure two more times, using each towelette or cotton ball only once. Maintains retraction of the foreskin until the specimen is obtained.			
5. Picks up the sterile specimen container and holds it near the meatus. Instructs the patient to begin voiding.			
6. Allows a small stream of urine to pass; and then without stopping the urine stream, places the specimen container into the stream, collecting approximately 30–60 mL.			
7. Removes the container from the stream, and allows the patient to finish emptying his bladder. *Note*: If the penis is uncircumcised, replaces the foreskin over the glans when the procedure is finished.			
8. Carefully replaces the sterile container lid, touching only the outside of the cap and container. Avoids touching the rim of the cup to the genital area. Does not get toilet paper, feces, pubic hair, menstrual blood, or anything else in the urine sample.			
9. Labels the container with the correct patient information (in many institutions, labels are preprinted or bar-coded). Places the container in a facility-specific carrier (usually a plastic bag) for transport to the lab.			
10. Removes gloves and washes hands. If the specimen has been obtained from a patient on a bedpan, leaves gloves on until it is removed, emptied, and stored properly.			
11. Assists patient back to bed.			
12. Transports the specimen to the lab in a timely manner.			

Recommendation: Pass _____ Needs more practice _____

Student: _____   Date: _____

Instructor: _____   Date: _____

PROCEDURE CHECKLIST
Chapter 28: Removing an Indwelling Catheter

Check (✓) Yes or No

PROCEDURE STEPS	Yes	No	COMMENTS
Before, during, and after the procedure, follows Principles-Based Checklist to Use With All Procedures, including: Identifies patient according to agency policy using two identifiers; attends appropriately to standard precautions, hand hygiene, safety, privacy, and body mechanics.			
1. Washes hands and dons clean procedure gloves.			
2. Instructs patient to assume a supine position.			
3. Places the catheter receptacle near patient (e.g., on the bed).			
4. Places a towel or waterproof drape between patient's legs and up by the urethral meatus.			
5. Obtains a sterile specimen (see Procedure for Obtaining a Clean Catch Urine Specimen), if needed. Some agencies require a culture and sensitivity test of the urine when an indwelling catheter is removed.			
6. Removes the device or tape securing the catheter to patient.			
7. Deflates the balloon completely by inserting a syringe into the balloon valve and allowing the balloon to self-deflate. Allows at least 30 seconds for the balloon to deflate. If aspiration is attempted, it is done slowly and gently. Verifies that the total fluid volume has been removed by checking the balloon size written on the valve port.			
8. If unable aspirate all the fluid, does not pull on the catheter. Reports to the change nurse or primary care provider before continuing the procedure.			
9. Instructs patient to relax and take a few deep breaths as the nurse slowly withdraws the catheter from the urethra.			
10. Wraps the catheter in the towel or drape.			
11. Uses warm water or perineal wash on gauze pads or perineal disposable wipes to cleanse the perineal area. A mild soap may also be used. Rinses well.			

PROCEDURE STEPS	Yes	No	COMMENTS
12. Measures the urine and then empties it in the toilet; discards the catheter, drainage tube, and collection bag in the biohazard waste receptacle.			
13. Explains to patient the need to monitor the first few voidings after catheter removal. If patient toilets independently, ask him to notify the nurse when he voids and to save the urine.			
14. Places a receptacle in the toilet or bedside commode if patient toilets independently.			
15. Removes and discards gloves; washes hands.			
16. Records the date and time of the procedure; the volume, color, and clarity of the urine; and the patient teaching.			

Recommendation: Pass _____ Needs more practice _____

Student: _____   Date: _____

Instructor: _____   Date: _____

PROCEDURE CHECKLIST
Chapter 29: Administering an Enema

Check (✓) Yes or No

PROCEDURE STEPS	Yes	No	COMMENTS
Administering Cleansing and Other Non-Prepackaged Enemas:			
Before, during, and after the procedure, follows Principles-Based Checklist to Use With All Procedures, including: Identifies the patient according to agency policy using two identifiers and attends appropriately to standard precautions, hand hygiene, safety, privacy, body mechanics, and documentation.			
1. Determines patient's ability to retain the enema solution.			
2. Places a bedpan or bedside commode nearby for patient with limited mobility.			
3. Opens the enema kit or obtains supplies.			
4. Warms the solution to 105°–110°F (40°–43°C), not in a microwave. Checks temperature with bath thermometer.			
5. Attaches tubing to the enema bucket if a bucket is being used. (The 1-L enema bag comes with preconnected tubing.)			
6. Closes the clamp on the tubing and fills the container with 500–1100 mL of warm solution (50–150 mL for infants; 250–350 mL for toddlers; 300–500 mL for school-age children).			
7. Adds castile soap or soap solution used by the facility, if a soapsuds enema was prescribed.			
8. Hangs the container on the IV pole.			
9. Holding the end of the tubing over a sink or waste can, opens the clamp and slowly allows the tubing to prime (fill) with solution. Reclamps when filled.			
10. Dons clean procedure gloves.			
11. Asks or assists patient to turn to a left side-lying position with the right knee flexed. (Elevates head of the bed very slightly for patients who have shortness of breath.)			
12. Places a waterproof pad under patient's buttocks/hips.			
13. Drapes patient with bath blanket, leaving only the buttocks and rectum exposed.			
14. Places the bedpan flat on the bed directly beneath the rectum, up against patient's buttocks; or places the bedside commode near the bed.			

PROCEDURE STEPS	Yes	No	COMMENTS
15. Generously lubricates the tip of the enema tubing.			
16. If necessary, lifts the superior buttock to expose the anus.			
17. Slowly and gently inserts tip of the tubing approximately 7–10 cm (3–4 in.) into the rectum; asks patient to take slow, deep breaths during this step.			
18. If tube does not pass with ease, does not force; allows a small amount of fluid to infuse and then tries again.			
19. Removes the container from the IV pole and holds it at the level of patient's hips. Begins instilling the solution.			
20. Slowly raises the level of the container so that it is 30–45 cm (12–18 in.) above the level of the hips. Adjusts the IV pole and rehangs the container.			
21. Continues a slow, steady instillation of the enema solution.			
22. Continuously monitors patient for pain or discomfort. If pain occurs or resistance is met at any time during the procedure, stops and consults with the primary care provider.			
23. Assesses ability to retain the solution. If patient has difficulty with retention, lowers the level of the container, stops the flow for 15–30 seconds, and then resumes the procedure.			
24. When the correct amount of solution has been instilled, clamps the tubing and slowly removes the tubing from the rectum.			
25. If there is stool on the tubing, wraps the end of the tubing in a disposable wipe or toilet tissue until it can be rinsed or disposed of.			
26. Cleanses patient's rectal area.			
27. Covers patient.			
28. Instructs patient to hold the enema solution for 5–15 minutes.			
29. Places the call light within reach.			
30. Disposes of enema supplies or, if reusable, cleans and stores in an appropriate location in patient's room.			
31. Removes gloves; performs hand hygiene.			
32. Depending on patient's mobility, assists onto the bedpan, to the bedside commode, or to the toilet when she feels compelled to defecate.			

PROCEDURE STEPS	Yes	No	COMMENTS
33. After patient has defecated, inspects the stool for color, consistency, and quantity.			
Administering a Prepackaged Enema:			
1. Determines patient's ability to retain the enema solution.			
2. Places a bedpan or bedside commode nearby for patient with limited mobility.			
3. Warms the solution—not in a microwave.			
4. Dons clean procedure gloves.			
5. Asks patient to turn or assists to turn to a left side-lying position with the right knee flexed. (Elevates head of the bed very slightly for patients who have shortness of breath.)			
6. Places a waterproof pad under patient's buttocks/hips.			
7. Drapes patient with bath blanket, leaving only the buttocks and rectum exposed.			
8. Opens the prepackaged enema. Removes the plastic cap from the container. The tip of the prepackaged enema container comes prelubricated. Adds extra lubricant as needed.			
9. If necessary, lifts the superior buttock to expose the anus.			
10. Slowly and gently inserts tip of the tubing approximately 7–10 cm (3–4 in.) into the rectum; asks patient to take slow, deep breaths during this step.			
11. If tube does not insert with ease, does not force; removes, relubricates, and retries.			
12. Tilts container slightly and slowly rolls and squeezes the container until all of the solution is instilled.			
13. Withdraws container tip from the rectum; wipes the area with a disposable wipe or toilet tissue.			
14. Covers patient and instructs to hold the enema solution for approximately 5–10 minutes.			
15. Disposes of empty container.			
16. Removes gloves; performs hand hygiene.			
17. Places the call light within reach.			
18. Depending on patient's mobility, assists onto the bedpan, to the bedside commode, or to the toilet when she feels compelled to defecate.			

PROCEDURE STEPS	Yes	No	COMMENTS
19. After patient has defecated, inspects the stool for color, consistency, and quantity.			
Administering an Oil-Retention Enema			
1. Obtains a commercial oil-retention enema kit.			
2. Warms the oil to body temperature by running warm tap water over the container. Tests a drop on arm.			
3. Dons clean procedure gloves.			
4. Asks patient to turn or assists to turn to a left side-lying position with the right knee flexed. (Elevates head of the bed very slightly for patients who have shortness of breath.)			
5. Places a waterproof pad under patient's buttocks/ hips.			
6. Drapes patient with bath blanket, leaving only the buttocks and rectum exposed.			
7. Opens the commercial oil-retention kit. Removes the plastic cap from the container. The tip of the prepackaged enema container comes prelubricated. Adds extra lubricant as needed.			
8. If necessary, lifts the superior buttock to expose the anus.			
9. Slowly and gently inserts tip of the tubing approximately 7–10 cm (3–4 in.) into the rectum; asks patient to take slow, deep breaths during this step.			
10. If tube does not insert with ease, does not force; removes, relubricates, and retries.			
11. Instills the oil into the rectum.			
12. Withdraws container tip from the rectum; wipes the area with a disposable wipe or toilet tissue.			
13. Covers patient and instructs to hold the enema solution for at least 30 minutes.			
14. Disposes of empty container.			
15. Removes gloves; performs hand hygiene.			
16. Places the call light within reach.			
17. Depending on patient's mobility, assists onto the bedpan, to the bedside commode, or to the toilet when she feels compelled to defecate.			
Administering a Return-Flow Enema:			
1. Obtains a rectal tube and solution container.			
2. Places a bedpan or bedside commode nearby for patient with limited mobility.			

PROCEDURE STEPS	Yes	No	COMMENTS
3. Prepares 100 to 200 mL tap water or saline. Warms the solution to 105°–110°F (40°–43°C), not in a microwave. Checks temperature with bath thermometer.			
4. Attaches tubing to the enema container and primes the tubing.			
5. Dons clean procedure gloves.			
6. Asks patient to turn or assists to turn to a left side-lying position with the right knee flexed. (Elevates head of the bed very slightly for patients who have shortness of breath.)			
7. Places a waterproof pad under patient's buttocks/hips.			
8. Drapes patient with bath blanket, leaving only the buttocks and rectum exposed.			
9. Generously lubricates the tip of the enema tubing.			
10. If necessary, lifts the superior buttock to expose the anus.			
11. Slowly and gently inserts the rectal tube approximately 7–10 cm (3–4 in.) into the rectum; asks patient to take slow, deep breaths during this step.			
12. If tube does not pass with ease, does not force; allows a small amount of fluid to infuse and then tries again.			
13. Holds the container at the level of patient's hips. Begins instilling the solution.			
14. Slowly raises the level of the container so that it is 30–45 cm (12–18 in.) above the level of the hips.			
15. Continues a slow, steady instillation of the enema solution.			
16. Instills all the solution into patient's rectum.			
17. When the correct amount of solution has been infused, lowers the tube and container below the level of the rectum and allows the solution to flow back into the container.			
18. Repeats instillation and return several times or until distention is relieved.			
19. Withdraws container tip from the rectum; wipes the area with a disposable wipe or toilet tissue.			
20. If there is stool on the tubing, wraps the end of the tubing in a disposable wipe or toilet tissue until it can be rinsed or disposed of.			
21. Removes gloves; performs hand hygiene.			
22. Places the call light within reach.			
23. Disposes of the empty container.			

PROCEDURE STEPS	Yes	No	COMMENTS

Recommendation: Pass _____ Needs more practice _____

Student: _____   Date: _____

Instructor: _____   Date: _____

250   Copyright © 2016, F. A. Davis Company, Wilkinson & Treas/Procedure Checklists for Fundamentals of Nursing, 3e

PROCEDURE CHECKLIST
Chapter 29: Changing an Ostomy Appliance

Check (✓) Yes or No

PROCEDURE STEPS	Yes	No	COMMENTS
Before, during, and after the procedure, follows Principles-Based Checklist to Use With All Procedures, including: Identifies the patient according to agency policy using two identifiers; attends appropriately to standard precautions, hand hygiene, safety, privacy, body mechanics, and documentation.			
1. Performs hand hygiene and dons clean procedure gloves.			
2. Folds down the linens to expose the ostomy site; places a clean towel across patient's abdomen under the existing pouch.			
3. Positions patient so that no skinfolds occur along the line of the stoma.			
4. If the pouch is drainable, opens it by removing the clamp and unrolling it at the bottom.			
5. Empties the existing ostomy pouch into a bedpan.			
6. Saves the clamp for reuse (note that some pouches cannot be drained).			
7. Using a silicone-based adhesive remover with one hand, uses the other hand to gently remove the old wafer from the skin, beginning at the top and proceeding in a downward direction.			
8. Places the old pouch and wafer in a plastic bag for disposal. If the pouch is nondrainable, disposes of it according to agency protocol.			
9. Inspects stoma and peristomal skin.			
10. Uses skin cleansing agent with a pH of 5.5 to cleanse stoma and surrounding skin.			
11. Allows the area to dry.			
12. Reports excess bleeding to the physician.			
13. Measures the size of the stoma in one of the following ways: a. Using a standard stoma measuring guide placed over the stoma			
b. Reusing a previously cut template			

PROCEDURE STEPS	Yes	No	COMMENTS
c. Measuring the stoma from side to side (approximating the circumference)			
14. Places a clean 4 in.×4 in. gauze pad over the stoma.			
15. Removes gloves and performs hand hygiene.			
16. Traces the size of the opening obtained in Step 13 onto the paper on the back of the new wafer; cuts the opening. Wafer opening is approximately 1.5–3 cm ($\frac{1}{16}$–$\frac{1}{8}$ in.) larger than the circumference of the stoma.			
17. Peels the paper off the wafer.			
18. *Note:* Some ostomy wafers come with an outer ring of tape attached. If so, does not remove the backing on this tape until the wafer is securely positioned (Steps 22–24).			
19. Dons clean procedure gloves.			
20. If ostomy skin care products are to be used, applies them at this time (e.g., wipes around stoma with skin-prep, applies skin barrier powder or paste, applies extra adhesive paste).			
21. Removes the gauze. Centers the wafer opening around the stoma and gently presses down. Presses hand firmly against the newly applied wafer and holds it for 30–60 seconds. a. *If using a one-piece pouch,* makes sure the bag is pointed toward patient's feet.			
b. *If using a two-piece system*, places the wafer on first. When the seal is complete, attaches the bag following manufacturer's instructions.			
c. *For an open-ended pouch*, folds the end of the pouch over the clamp and closes the clamp, listening for a "click" to ensure it is secure.			
22. Removes gloves and performs hand hygiene.			
23. Returns patient to a comfortable position.			
24. Disposes of used ostomy pouch following agency policy for biohazardous waste.			

Recommendation: Pass _____ Needs more practice _____

Student: _____ Date: _____

Instructor: _____ Date: _____

 Copyright © 2016, F. A. Davis Company, Wilkinson & Treas/Procedure Checklists for Fundamentals of Nursing, 3e

PROCEDURE CHECKLIST
Chapter 29: Inserting a Rectal Tube

Check (✓) Yes or No

PROCEDURE STEPS	Yes	No	COMMENTS
Before, during, and after the procedure, follows Principles-Based Checklist to Use With All Procedures, including: Identifies the patient according to agency policy using two identifiers; attends appropriately to standard precautions, hand hygiene, safety, privacy, body mechanics, and documentation.			
1. Dons procedure gloves.			
2. Asks patient to lift hips or roll from side to side to place a waterproof pad.			
3. Attaches a collecting device to the end of the rectal tube: Tapes a plastic bag or urine collection bag around the distal end of the rectal tube and vents the upper side of the bag; or inserts the tube into the specimen container; or places the end of the tube in a graduated container partially filled with water.			
4. Places patient in left side-lying position. Drapes for privacy.			
5. Lubricates the tip of the rectal tube.			
6. Separates the buttocks, asks patient to take a deep breath, and gently inserts the tube into the rectum. Adults: 10–12.5 cm (4–5 in.); children: 5–10 cm (2–4 in.).			
7. For adults, tapes the tube in place; for children, holds it manually.			
8. Leaves the rectal tube in place for 15–20 minutes. If distention persists, reinserts the tube every 2–3 hours.			
9. Assists patient to move about in bed to promote gas expulsion. A knee–chest position is ideal.			
10. Removes the tube, wipes the buttocks with tissue, and assists to clean the rectal area as needed.			
11. Disposes of used equipment, or cleans it if it is to be reused.			

Recommendation: Pass _____ Needs more practice _____

Student: _____ Date: _____

Instructor: _____ Date: _____

PROCEDURE CHECKLIST
Chapter 29: Irrigating a Colostomy

Check (✔) Yes or No

PROCEDURE STEPS	Yes	No	COMMENTS
Before, during, and after the procedure, follows Principles-Based Checklist to Use With All Procedures, including: Identifies the patient according to agency policy using two identifiers; attends appropriately to standard precautions, hand hygiene, safety, privacy, body mechanics, and documentation.			
1. Places the IV pole near where the procedure will take place (e.g., in the bathroom or next to the bed).			
2. Assists patient to the bathroom (if possible).			
3. Asks patient if she prefers to sit directly on the toilet or on a chair in front of it.			
4. If patient must remain in bed, elevates the head of the bed.			
5. Prepares the irrigation container. a. For two-piece systems, connects the tubing to the container.			
b. Clamps the tubing. Fills the container with 500–1000 mL of warm tap water.			
6. Primes the tubing; unclamps the tubing to allow for filling.			
7. Hangs the solution container on the IV pole. Adjusts the pole to the height of patient's shoulder (approximately 45 cm [18 in.] above the stoma).			
8. Performs hand hygiene and dons clean procedure gloves.			
9. Removes the existing colostomy appliance following the steps in Procedure Checklist Chapter 29: Changing an Ostomy Appliance.			
10. Disposes of the used colostomy appliance properly. Empties contents into bedpan or toilet and discards the pouch in a moisture-proof (e.g., plastic) bag.			
11. Inspects the stoma and surrounding skin area.			
12. Applies the colostomy irrigation sleeve, following the manufacturer's directions. a. *Sleeves with adhesive backing* are applied following pouch application steps found in Procedure Checklist Chapter 29: Changing an Ostomy Appliance.			
b. *Sleeves without an adhesive backing*: Places the belt around patient's waist and attaches the ends to the pouch flange on either side.			
c. For patients sitting in front of the toilet or commode, places a waterproof pad under the sleeve over the thighs.			

Copyright © 2016, F. A. Davis Company, Wilkinson & Treas/Procedure Checklists for Fundamentals of Nursing, 3e

PROCEDURE STEPS	Yes	No	COMMENTS
13. *Note:* For patients sitting directly on a toilet or commode, the end of the sleeve should hang down past patient's pubic area, but not into the water. For a patient in bed, places the end of the sleeve in the bedpan.			
14. Generously lubricates the cone at the end of the irrigation tubing with water-soluble lubricant.			
15. Opens the top of the irrigation sleeve; inserts the cone gently into the colostomy stoma and holds it solidly in place.			
16. Opens the clamp on the tubing and slowly begins the flow of water. The fluid should flow in at a rate of about 1 liter per 5–10 minutes, or as patient can tolerate.			
17. If patient complains of discomfort, stops the flow for 15–30 seconds and asks patient to take deep breaths.			
18. When the correct amount of solution has instilled, clamps the tubing and removes the cone from the stoma.			
19. Wraps the end of the cone in tissue or paper towel until it can be cleaned or disposed of properly.			
20. Closes the top of the irrigation sleeve with a clamp.			
21. Instructs patient to remain sitting until most of the irrigation fluid and bowel contents have evacuated. *Note:* Can also clamp the end of the sleeve and ask patient to ambulate to stimulate complete evacuation of stool. Or instructs patient to massage the abdomen.			
22. When evacuation is complete, opens the top clamp, and rinses and removes the irrigation sleeve. Sets it aside.			
23. Cleanses the stoma and peristomal area with a warm prepackaged disposable wipe; allows to dry.			
24. Preps the skin and applies a new colostomy appliance, if patient is wearing one, following the steps in Procedure Checklist Chapter 29: Changing an Ostomy Appliance. Otherwise, covers the stoma with a small gauze bandage.			
25. Cleans the irrigation sleeve with mild soap and water. Allows it to dry.			
26. Places the irrigation supplies in the proper place (e.g., in a plastic container or plastic bag).			
27. Removes gloves and performs hand hygiene.			
28. Assists patient back to a position of comfort.			

Recommendation: Pass _____ Needs more practice _____

Student: _____ Date: _____

Instructor: _____ Date: _____

 Copyright © 2016, F. A. Davis Company, Wilkinson & Treas/Procedure Checklists for Fundamentals of Nursing, 3e

PROCEDURE CHECKLIST
Chapter 29: Placing and Removing a Bedpan

Check (✓) Yes or No

PROCEDURE STEPS	Yes	No	COMMENTS
Before, during, and after the procedure, follows Principles-Based Checklist to Use With All Procedures, including: Identifies the patient according to agency policy using two identifiers; attends appropriately to standard precautions, hand hygiene, safety, privacy, body mechanics, and documentation.			
1. Determines whether patient needs regular bedpan or fracture pan.			
2. Obtains and takes the necessary supplies to patient's room. Leaves packet of prepackaged disposable wipes at the bedside for use during bedpan removal.			
3. If the bedpan is metal, places it under warm, running water for a few seconds; then dries, making sure the bedpan is not too hot.			
4. Raises siderail on the opposite side of the bed.			
5. Raises the bed to a comfortable working height.			
6. Prepares patient by folding down the covers to a point that will allow placement of the bedpan, yet expose only as much of her body as necessary.			
7. Performs hand hygiene and dons clean procedure gloves.			
8. Notes the presence of dressings, drains, intravenous fluids, and traction and ensures there is a linen-saver pad in place.			
For Patients Who Are Able to Move/Turn Independently in Bed:			
9. Ask for help, if needed. Places patient supine; lowers the head of the bed.			
10. Prepares patient to position the bedpan. a. Asks patient to lift his hips. Patient may need to raise his knees to a flexed position, place his feet flat on the bed and push up. Slides a hand under the small of patient's back, as needed, to assist patient.			
b. Alternatively, places patient in a semi-Fowler's position; asks him to raise his hips by pushing up on raised siderails or by using an overbed trapeze.			
11. Places the bedpan under patient's buttocks with the wide, rounded end toward the back. When using a fracture pan, places the wide, rounded end toward the front.			
12. Avoids sliding the pan against the patient's skin.			

PROCEDURE STEPS	Yes	No	COMMENTS
13. Repositions patient:			
a. Replaces the covers; raises the head of the bed to a position of comfort for patient.			
b. Places a rolled towel, blanket, or small pillow under the sacrum (lumbar curve of the back).			
c. Places the call light and toilet tissue within patient's reach.			
d. Places bed back in its lowest position and raises both upper siderails.			
14. Removes gloves and washes hands.			
For Patients Who Are Unable to Move/Turn Independently:			
15. Asks for help from another healthcare worker, as needed.			
16. With patient supine, lowers the head of the bed.			
17. Assists patient to a side-lying position, using a turning sheet if necessary.			
18. Places the bedpan up against patient's buttocks with the wide, rounded end toward the head. When using a fracture pan, places the wide rounded end toward the feet.			
19. Holding the bedpan in place, slowly rolls patient back and onto the bedpan.			
20. Repositions patient:			
a. Replaces the covers; raises the head of the bed to a position of comfort for patient.			
b. Places a rolled towel, blanket, or small pillow under the sacrum (lumbar curve of the back).			
c. Places the call light and toilet tissue within patient's reach.			
d. Places bed back in its lowest position and raises both upper siderails.			
21. Removes gloves and washes hands.			
Removing the Bedpan:			
22. Dons clean procedure gloves.			
23. Opens the prepackaged disposable wipes and places near the work area.			
24. If patient is immobile, lowers head of bed; raises bed to comfortable working height.			
25. Pulls covers down only as far as necessary to remove the bedpan.			
26. Offers patient toilet paper (assists as needed).			

PROCEDURE STEPS	Yes	No	COMMENTS
27. Asks patient to raise her hips. Stabilizes and removes the bedpan. If patient is unable to raise her hips, stabilizes the bedpan and assists her to the side-lying position.			
28. Cleanses the buttocks with a prepackaged disposable wipe and allows to air dry.			
29. Replaces covers and positions patient for comfort.			
30. Offers the second warm, prepackaged disposable wipe to patient to cleanse her hands.			
31. Empties the bedpan in patient's toilet.			
32. Measures output if I&O is part of the treatment plan.			
33. Cleans bedpan following facility guidelines.			
34. Removes soiled gloves and performs hand hygiene.			

Recommendation: Pass _____ Needs more practice _____

Student: _____   Date: _____

Instructor: _____   Date: _____

PROCEDURE CHECKLIST
Chapter 29: Placing Fecal Drainage Devices

Check (✓) Yes or No

PROCEDURE STEPS	Yes	No	COMMENTS
Before, during, and after the procedure, follows Principles-Based Checklist to Use With All Procedures, including: Identifies the patient according to agency policy using two identifiers; attends appropriately to standard precautions, hand hygiene, safety, privacy, body mechanics, and documentation.			
1. Obtains assistance as needed.			
2. Dons procedure gloves.			
3. Places patient in left side-lying position.			
4. Drapes to expose the buttocks.			
5. Cleanses perineal area; dries well.			
6. Trims perianal hair, if present.			
7. Wipes the area with skin protectant wipes.			
8. Spreads buttocks to expose rectum.			
9. Removes the backing from the adhesive on the fecal bag, and applies it, placing opening over the anus, and avoiding gaps and creases.			
10. Releases buttocks.			
11. Connects incontinence pouch to a drainage bat.			
12. Hangs drainage bag below level of patient.			
Inserting an Indwelling Fecal Drainage Device:			
1. Ensures that a primary care provider has performed a digital rectal exam.			
2. Dons procedure gloves, mask, and goggles.			
3. Places patient in left side-lying position.			
4. Removes any indwelling device.			
5. Depending on the type of device, verifies proper inflation and deflation of the intralumenal balloon: Attaches syringe, inflates with recommended amount of air, deflates, and removes syringe.			

PROCEDURE STEPS	Yes	No	COMMENTS
6. Depending on the device, fills the retention cuff with 35–40 mL of water; disconnects the syringe and checks for leaks. After verifying function, slowly and completely aspirates all fluid from cuff and balloon and disconnects the syringe.			
7. Connects the indwelling tube to the collection bag. Clamps and hangs the bag lower than the level of patient.			
8. If the system has an "introducer," inflates with air through the connector on the tube; disconnects the syringe.			
9. Inserts a lubricated, gloved index finger into the balloon cuff finger pocket (located above the position indicator line) and coats the balloon generously with lubricant.			
10. Gently inserts the balloon end of the catheter through the anal sphincter until the balloon is beyond the anus and well inside the rectal vault.			
11. Inflates the retention cuff with water or saline per the manufacturer's guidelines. Does not overfill.			
12. Removes the syringe from the inflation port and puts gentle traction on the catheter.			
13. If an intralumenal balloon or introducer was inflated in Step 8, completely aspirates the air from it now.			
14. Does not leave patient unattended while the intralumenal balloon is inflated.			
15. If the device has anchoring straps, applies protective skin care dressing and tapes one strap to each buttock.			
16. Positions tubing along patient's leg, avoiding kinks and obstruction; positions collection bag lower than patient.			
17. Disposes of used equipment and washes hands.			

Recommendation: Pass _____ Needs more practice _____

Student: _____   Date: _____

Instructor: _____   Date: _____

Check (✓) Yes or No

PROCEDURE STEPS	Yes	No	COMMENTS
Before, during, and after the procedure, follows Principles-Based Checklist to Use With All Procedures, including: Identifies the patient according to agency policy using two identifiers; attends appropriately to standard precautions, hand hygiene, safety, privacy, body mechanics, and documentation.			
1. Trims and files own fingernails if they extend over the end of the fingertips.			
2. Obtains baseline vital signs and determines whether patient has a history of cardiac problems or other contraindications.			
3. Checks to see if an oil retention enema is prescribed before and/or after the procedure. Administers, if so.			
4. Obtains correct lubricant (e.g., Lidocaine, if ordered).			
5. Drapes patient to expose only the rectal area.			
6. Assists patient to turn to his left side with his right knee flexed toward his head.			
7. Places a waterproof pad halfway beneath the left hip.			
8. Dons clean procedure gloves; double gloves if desired or if dictated by policy.			
9. Exposes patient's buttocks; places a clean, dry bedpan on the waterproof pad, next to the buttocks.			
10. Opens packet of prepackaged disposable wipes or places toilet tissue nearby to cleanse the rectal area upon completion of the procedure.			
11. Generously lubricates the gloved forefinger and/or middle finger of the dominant hand.			
12. Slowly slides one lubricated finger into the rectum. Observes for perianal irritation.			
13. Gently rotates the finger around the mass and/or into the mass.			
14. Begins to break the stool into smaller pieces. One method is to insert a second finger and gently "slice" apart the stool using a scissoring motion. Removes pieces of stool as they become separated, and places them in the bedpan.			

PROCEDURE STEPS	Yes	No	COMMENTS
15. Instructs patient to take slow, deep breaths during the procedure.			
16. Allowing patient to rest at intervals, continues to manipulate and remove pieces of stool.			
17. Reapplies lubricant each time fingers are reinserted.			
18. Assesses patient's heart rate at regular intervals. Stops the procedure if heart rate falls or rhythm changes from the initial assessment.			
19. Depending on agency policy and nursing judgment, limits session to four finger insertions and gives a suppository between subsequent sessions.			
20. When removal of stool is complete, covers bedpan and sets aside.			
21. Uses prepackaged disposable wipe and/or toilet tissue to cleanse the rectal area.			
22. Assists patient to a position of comfort.			
23. Notes color, amount, and consistency of stool.			
24. Disposes of stool and cleans bedpan properly.			
25. Removes gloves and performs hand hygiene.			

Recommendation: Pass _____ Needs more practice _____

Student: _____   Date: _____

Instructor: _____   Date: _____

PROCEDURE CHECKLIST
Chapter 29: Testing Stool for Occult Blood

Check (✓) Yes or No

PROCEDURE STEPS	Yes	No	COMMENTS
Before, during, and after the procedure, follows Principles-Based Checklist to Use With All Procedures, including: Identifies the patient according to agency policy and two identifiers; attends appropriately to standard precautions, hand hygiene, safety, privacy, body mechanics, and documentation.			
1. Determines whether the test will be done by the nurse at the point of care or by lab personnel.			
2. Gathers the necessary testing supplies.			
3. Instructs patient to void before collecting the stool specimen.			
4. Performs hand hygiene and dons procedure gloves.			
5. Places a clean, dry container for the stool specimen into the toilet or bedside commode in such a manner that the urine falls into the toilet and the fecal specimen falls into the container. Obtains a clean, dry bedpan for patient who is immobile.			
6. Instructs patient to defecate into the container, or places patient on the bedpan.			
7. Does not contaminate the specimen with toilet tissue.			
8. Once the specimen has been obtained and the bedpan removed (or patient assisted to bed), performs hand hygiene and dons clean procedure gloves.			
9. Explains the purpose of the test and that serial specimens may be needed.			
10. Reads the directions for the testing kit.			
11. Opens the specimen side of the fecal occult blood test slide. With a wooden tongue depressor or other applicator, collects a small sample of stool and spreads thinly onto one "window" of the slide.			
12. Uses a different applicator or the opposite end of the depressor to collect a second small sample of stool.			
13. Spreads the second sample thinly onto the second "window" of the slide.			
14. Wraps depressor in tissue and paper towel; places in waste receptacle. Does not flush it.			
15. Closes the fecal occult blood test slide.			

PROCEDURE STEPS	Yes	No	COMMENTS
16. If the test is to be done by laboratory personnel, labels the specimen properly and places into the proper receptacle for transportation to the lab.			
17. If test is to be done at the bedside, turns the slide over and opens the opposite side of the package.			
18. Follows the directions on the package regarding the number of drops of the developing solution.			
19. Follows package directions for interpreting test results.			
20. Removes gloves and performs hand hygiene.			

Recommendation: Pass _____ Needs more practice _____

Student: _____   Date: _____

Instructor: _____   Date: _____

PROCEDURE CHECKLIST
Chapter 30: Performing Otic Irrigation

Check (✓) Yes or No

PROCEDURE STEPS	Yes	No	COMMENTS
Before, during, and after the procedure, follows Principles-Based Checklist to Use With All Procedures, including: Identifies the patient according to agency policy; attends appropriately to standard precautions, hand hygiene, safety, privacy, and body mechanics.			
1. Warms the irrigating solution to body temperature (98.6°F [37°C]) and fills the reservoir of the irrigator.			
2. Assembles irrigator, if necessary, and places a clean disposable tip on it.			
3. Assists the client into a sitting or lying position with the head tilted away from the affected ear.			
4. Dons gloves; puts on headlight.			
5. Drapes the client with a plastic drape and places a towel on the client's shoulder on the side being irrigated.			
6. Has the client hold an emesis basin under the ear. *Note:* An emesis basin is not necessary if a comprehensive ear wash system is used.			
7. If using an ear wash system, flushes the system for 20–30 seconds to remove air. If using an Asepto or rubber bulb syringe, fills the syringe with about 50 mL of the irrigating solution, and expels any remaining air.			
8. Straightens the ear canal. a. For a child younger than 3 years old, pulls the pinna down and back.			
b. For older children and adults, pulls the pinna upward and outward.			
9. Instructs patient to indicate if any pain or dizziness occurs during the irrigation.			
10. Explains to patient that he may feel warmth, fullness, or pressure when the fluid reaches the tympanic membrane.			
11. Places the tip of the nozzle (or syringe) about 1 cm (½ in.) above the entrance of the ear canal and directs the stream of irrigating solution gently along the top of the ear canal toward the back of patient's head.			
12. Does not occlude the ear canal with the nozzle.			
13. Instills the solution slowly.			

PROCEDURE STEPS	Yes	No	COMMENTS
14. Allows the solution to flow out as it is instilled.			
15. Repeats Steps 11–14 for 5 minutes or until cerumen appears in the return solution.			
16. Inspects the ear with an otoscope to evaluate cerumen removal. Continues irrigating until the canal is cleaned.			
17. Places a cotton ball loosely in the ear canal and instructs patient to lie on the side of the affected ear.			
18. Cleans and disinfects the irrigator according to the manufacturer's instructions or agency protocols.			
19. Disposes of disposable tips and other supplies.			

Recommendation: Pass _____ Needs more practice _____

Student: _____   Date: _____

Instructor: _____   Date: _____

 Copyright © 2016, F. A. Davis Company, Wilkinson & Treas/Procedure Checklists for Fundamentals of Nursing, 3e

PROCEDURE CHECKLIST
Chapter 31: Setting Up and Managing Patient-Controlled Analgesia by Pump

Check (✓) Yes or No

PROCEDURE STEPS	Yes	No	COMMENTS
Before, during, and after the procedure, follows Principles-Based Checklist to Use With All Procedures, including: Identifies the patient according to agency policy; attends appropriately to standard precautions, hand hygiene, safety, privacy, and body mechanics.			
1. Initiates IV therapy if patient does not have an IV solution infusing.			
2. Obtains and double-checks medication with the original prescription.			
3. Double-checks dose calculation.			
4. Removes air from the vial or cartridge.			
5. Connects PCA tubing to the vial or cartridge.			
6. Determines (calculates if necessary) the: a. On-demand dose			
b. Lock-out interval			
c. Basal rate			
d. One-time bolus (loading) dose			
e. The 1-hour or 4-hour lock-out interval			
7. Calculates correct settings as prescribed.			
8. Primes the tubing up to the Y-connector; then clamps the tubing above the connector.			
9. Inserts the cartridge or vial injector into the pump and locks the pump; or follows the manufacturer's instruction manual.			
10. Turns the pump on and sets the parameters (listed in Step 6a through e) according to the prescriptions and own calculations.			
11. Scrubs the port on the IV tubing closest to patient with alcohol or chlorhexidine-alcohol–based product and connects the PCA pump tubing.			
12. Opens the clamp and starts the pump.			

PROCEDURE STEPS	Yes	No	COMMENTS
13. Administers the bolus (loading) dose if prescribed. Remains present with patient as the dose is delivered.			
14. Closes the pump door and locks the machine with the key.			
15. Checks for flashing lights or alarms that may indicate the need to correct settings.			
16. Makes sure tubing clamps are released, and presses the start button to begin the pump operation.			
17. Puts the control button for on-demand doses within patient's reach making sure the PCA cord is placed away from the call bell.			

Recommendation: Pass _____ Needs more practice _____

Student: _____   Date: _____

Instructor: _____   Date: _____

PROCEDURE CHECKLIST
Chapter 32: Assisting With Ambulation (One Nurse)

Check (✓) Yes or No

PROCEDURE STEPS	Yes	No	COMMENTS
Before, during, and after the procedure, follows Principles-Based Checklist to Use With All Procedures, including: Identifies the patient according to agency policy; attends appropriately to standard precautions, hand hygiene, safety, privacy, and body mechanics.			
1. Puts nonskid footwear on patient.			
2. Places the bed in a low position and locks the wheels.			
3. Applies a transfer belt.			
4. Assists patient to dangle at the side of the bed. (See Procedure Checklist Chapter 32: Dangling a Patient at the Side of the Bed.)			
5. Faces patient. Braces feet and knees against patient's feet and knees, paying particular attention to any known weakness.			
6. Bends from the hips and knees, and holds onto the transfer belt.			
7. Instructs patient to place her arms around the nurse between the shoulders and waist (the location depends on the nurse's height and the height of patient).			
8. Asks patient to stand as the nurse moves to an upright position by straightening the legs and hips.			
9. Allows patient to steady herself for a moment.			
10. Stands at patient's side, placing both hands on the transfer belt.			
11. If patient has weakness on one side, positions self on the weaker side.			
12. Slowly guides patient forward, observing for signs of fatigue or dizziness.			
13. If patient must transport an IV pole, allows patient to hold onto the pole on the side where the nurse is standing. Assists patient to advance the pole as patient ambulates.			

Recommendation: Pass _____ Needs more practice _____

Student: _____ Date: _____

Instructor: _____ Date: _____

Copyright © 2016, F. A. Davis Company, Wilkinson & Treas/Procedure Checklists for Fundamentals of Nursing, 3e

PROCEDURE CHECKLIST
Chapter 32: Assisting With Ambulation (Two Nurses)

Check (✓) Yes or No

PROCEDURE STEPS	Yes	No	COMMENTS
Before, during, and after the procedure, follows Principles-Based Checklist to Use With All Procedures, including: Identifies the patient according to agency policy; attends appropriately to standard precautions, hand hygiene, safety, privacy, and body mechanics.			
1. Puts nonskid footwear on patient.			
2. Places the bed in a low position.			
3. Locks bed wheels.			
4. Applies a transfer belt.			
5. Assists patient to dangle at the side of the bed. (See Procedure Checklist Chapter 32: Dangling a Patient at the Side of the Bed.)			
6. Each nurse stands facing patient on opposite sides of patient, bracing their feet and knees against patient's, and paying particular attention to any known weakness.			
7. Bends from the hips and knees, and holds onto the transfer belt.			
8. Instructs patient to place her arms around each of the nurses between the shoulders and waist (the location depends on the nurses' height and the height of patient).			
9. Asks patient to stand as the nurses move to an upright position by straightening their legs and hips.			
10. Allows patient to steady herself for a moment.			
11. Both nurses stand at patient's sides, grasping hold of the transfer belt.			
12. Slowly guides patient forward, observing for fatigue or dizziness.			
13. If patient must transport an IV pole, one nurse advances the IV pole along the side of patient by holding the pole with the outside hand.			

Recommendation: Pass _____ Needs more practice _____

Student: _____   Date: _____

Instructor: _____   Date: _____

Copyright © 2016, F. A. Davis Company, Wilkinson & Treas/Procedure Checklists for Fundamentals of Nursing, 3e

Check (✓) Yes or No

PROCEDURE STEPS	Yes	No	COMMENTS
Before, during, and after the procedure, follows Principles-Based Checklist to Use With All Procedures, including: Identifies the patient according to agency policy; attends appropriately to standard precautions, hand hygiene, safety, privacy, and body mechanics.			
1. Locks bed wheels.			
2. Places patient in supine position and raises the head of the bed to 90°.			
3. Keeps siderail elevated on the side opposite where the nurse is standing.			
4. Applies a gait transfer belt to patient at waist level.			
5. Places the bed in a low position.			
6. Stands at the side of the bed, facing patient, with a wide base of support. Places foot closest to the head of the bed forward of the other foot. Leans forward, bending at the hips with the knees flexed.			
7. Positions hands on either side of the gait transfer belt.			
8. Rocks onto the back foot while moving patient into a sitting position on the side of the bed—by pulling patient by the gait transfer belt.			
9. Stays with patient as he dangles.			
10. Reassesses comfort level and for dizziness.			

Recommendation: Pass _____ Needs more practice _____

Student: _____   Date: _____

Instructor: _____   Date: _____

PROCEDURE CHECKLIST
Chapter 32: Logrolling a Patient

Check (✔) Yes or No

PROCEDURE STEPS	Yes	No	COMMENTS
Before, during, and after the procedure, follows Principles-Based Checklist to Use With All Procedures, including: Identifies the patient according to agency policy; attends appropriately to standard precautions, hand hygiene, safety, privacy, and body mechanics.			
1. Locks the bed.			
2. Lowers the head of the bed and places patient supine.			
3. Lowers the siderail on the side where the nurse is standing; keeps rail up on opposite side.			
4. Raises height of the bed to waist level.			
5. Ensures that a friction-reducing device such as a transfer roller sheet is in place; improvises with a plastic bag or film under patient, if needed.			
6. Positions one staff member at patient's head and shoulders, responsible for moving the head and neck as a unit. Positions the other person at patient's hips. If three staff members are needed, positions one at the shoulders, one at the waist, and the third at thigh level.			
7. Each nurse positions her feet with a wide base of support, with one foot slightly more forward than the other.			
8. Uses a drawsheet to move patient to the side of the bed on which the nurses are standing.			
9. Positions patient's head with a pillow.			
10. Instructs patient to fold her arms across her chest.			
11. Places a pillow between patient's knees.			
12. One nurse always supports the head and shoulders during the move. The move is smooth so that the head and hips are kept in alignment.			
13. Raises siderail and moves to the opposite side of the bed.			
14. Lowers siderail on the "new" side and faces patient.			
15. All nurses flex their knees and hips, and shift their weight to the back foot on the count of three, being sure to support head as patient is rolled.			
16. Places pillows to maintain patient in a lateral position.			

PROCEDURE STEPS	Yes	No	COMMENTS
17. Places bed in low position and raises siderails.			
18. Places call device within reach.			

Recommendation: Pass _____ Needs more practice _____

Student: _____   Date: _____

Instructor: _____   Date: _____

278   Copyright © 2016, F. A. Davis Company, Wilkinson & Treas/Procedure Checklists for Fundamentals of Nursing, 3e

PROCEDURE CHECKLIST
Chapter 32: Moving a Patient Up in Bed

Check (✓) Yes or No

PROCEDURE STEPS	Yes	No	COMMENTS
Before, during, and after the procedure, follows Principles-Based Checklist to Use With All Procedures, including: Identifies the patient according to agency policy; attends appropriately to standard precautions, hand hygiene, safety, privacy, and body mechanics.			
1. Medicates the patient for pain, if needed, before moving up in bed.			
2. Obtains the help of a second person to move patient.			
3. Locks the bed wheels.			
4. Lowers the head of the bed; places patient supine.			
5. Lowers siderail on "working" side; keeps siderail up on opposite side of the bed.			
6. Raises the height of the bed to waist level.			
7. Ensures that a friction-reducing device such as a transfer roller sheet is in place; improvises with a plastic bag or film under patient, if needed.			
8. Removes the pillow from under patient's head and places it at the head of the bed.			
9. Instructs patient to fold his arms across his chest. If an overhead trapeze is in place, asks patient to hold the trapeze with both hands. Has patient bend his knees with feet flat on the bed.			
10. Instructs patient to flex his neck.			
11. Positions the assistant on the opposite side of bed; each grasps and rolls the drawsheet close to patient.			
12. Instructs patient, on the count of three, to lift his trunk and push off with his heels toward the head of the bed.			
13. Positions own feet with a wide base of support. Points the feet toward the direction of the move. Flexes own knees and hips.			
14. Places own weight on the foot nearest to the foot of the bed. Counts to three and shifts weight toward the head of the bed.			
15. Repeats until patient is positioned near the head of the bed.			
16. Straightens drawsheet, places a pillow under patient's head, and assists him to a comfortable position.			

PROCEDURE STEPS	Yes	No	COMMENTS
17. Places the bed in low position, and raises the siderail.			
18. Places the call device in a position where patient can easily reach it.			
Moving a Patient Using an Approved Mechanical Lifting Device:			
19. Locks the bed wheels, lowers the head of the bed, and places patient supine.			
20. Positions a nurse on each side of the bed.			
21. Lowers the siderails and raises height of bed to waist level.			
22. Uses the drawsheet to turn patient to one side.			
23. Positions the midline of the full body sling at the patient's back. Tightly rolls the remaining half and tucks it under the drawsheet.			
24. Uses the drawsheet to turn patient to the opposite side and unrolls the full body sling.			
25. Repositions the patient supine.			
26. Attaches the sling to the overbed lifting device or mechanical lift.			
27. Engages the lift to raise patient off of the bed. Advances the lift toward the head of the bed until patient is at the desired level.			
28. Lowers the lift and removes sling from underneath patient, if needed.			
29. Turns patient to the desired position. Straightens the drawsheet and tucks it in tightly at the sides of the bed.			

Recommendation: Pass _____ Needs more practice _____

Student: _____   Date: _____

Instructor: _____   Date: _____

PROCEDURE CHECKLIST
Chapter 32: Transferring a Patient From Bed to Chair

Check (✓) Yes or No

PROCEDURE STEPS	Yes	No	COMMENTS
Before, during, and after the procedure, follows Principles-Based Checklist to Use With All Procedures, including: Identifies the patient according to agency policy; attends appropriately to standard precautions, hand hygiene, safety, privacy, and body mechanics.			
1. Positions the chair next to the bed and near the head of the bed. If possible, locks the chair.			
2. Puts nonskid footwear on patient.			
3. Places the bed in a low position.			
4. Locks the bed wheels.			
5. Applies the transfer belt.			
6. Assists patient to dangle at the side of the bed. (See Procedure Checklist Chapter 32: Dangling a Patient at the Side of the Bed.)			
7. Stands toward the bed, facing patient; braces feet and knees against patient's legs. Pays particular attention to any known weakness.			
8. Bends hips and knees, keeps back straight, holds onto the transfer belt. If two nurses are available, one nurse should be on each side of patient.			
9. Instructs patient to place her arms around the nurse between the shoulders and waist (the exact location depends on the height of the nurse and patient).			
10. Asks patient to stand as the nurse moves to an upright position by straightening her legs and hips.			
11. Allows patient to steady herself for a moment.			
12. Instructs patient to pivot and turn with the nurse toward the chair.			
13. Assists patient to position herself in front of the chair and place her hands on the arms of the chair.			
14. Asks patient to flex her hips and knees as she lowers herself to the chair. Guides her motion while maintaining a firm hold of patient.			

15. Assists patient to a comfortable position in the chair. Provides a blanket, if needed.			
16. Places the call device within reach.			

Recommendation: Pass _____ Needs more practice _____

Student: _____   Date: _____

Instructor: _____   Date: _____

 Copyright © 2016, F. A. Davis Company, Wilkinson & Treas/Procedure Checklists for Fundamentals of Nursing, 3e

Chapter 32: Transferring a Patient From Bed to Stretcher

Check (✔) Yes or No

PROCEDURE STEPS	Yes	No	COMMENTS
Before, during, and after the procedure, follows Principles-Based Checklist to Use With All Procedures, including: Identifies the patient according to agency policy; attends appropriately to standard precautions, hand hygiene, safety, privacy, and body mechanics.			
1. Locks the bed wheels.			
2. Positions the bed flat (if patient can tolerate being supine) and at the height of the stretcher.			
3. Lowers the siderails.			
4. Positions at least one nurse on each side of the bed.			
5. Moves patient in supine position to the side of the bed where the stretcher will be placed by rolling up the drawsheet close to patient's body and pulling.			
6. Aligns patient's legs and head with her trunk.			
7. Positions stretcher next to the bed.			
8. Locks the stretcher wheels.			
9. Places a friction-reducing device over the transfer board.			
10. Nurse on the side of the bed opposite the stretcher uses drawsheet to turn patient away from the stretcher; the other nurse places the transfer board against patient's back, halfway between the bed and the stretcher.			
11. Turns patient onto her back and onto the transfer board, ensuring that her feet and shoulder are over the edge of the transfer board.			
12. Has patient raise her head, if able.			
13. Uses drawsheet to slide patient across the transfer board onto the stretcher.			
14. Turns patient away from the bed and removes the board and transfer roller sheet.			
15. Repositions patient on the stretcher for comfort and alignment; provides a blanket if needed.			
16. Fastens safety belts and raises stretcher siderails.			

PROCEDURE STEPS	Yes	No	COMMENTS
Variation: Transferring From Bed to Stretcher With a Slipsheet:			
17. Positions the bed flat, positions the patient supine, adjusts the stretcher height (as above).			
18. With the drawsheet, turns the patient to the side opposite where the stretcher will be placed.			
19. Positions the slipsheet under the patient by rolling the patient to one side and tucking the slipsheet under her.			
20. Turns patient to the opposite side and pulls the slipsheet from under patient.			
21. Places patient supine.			
22. Lowers the siderail on the side where the stretcher will be placed.			
23. Moves the stretcher next to the bed and locks the wheels.			
24. Positions at least two nurses on the far side of the stretcher. Pulls patient onto the stretcher by pulling on the slipsheet.			

Recommendation: Pass _____ Needs more practice _____

Student: _____ Date: _____

Instructor: _____ Date: _____

 Copyright © 2016, F. A. Davis Company, Wilkinson & Treas/Procedure Checklists for Fundamentals of Nursing, 3e

PROCEDURE CHECKLIST
Chapter 32: Turning a Patient in Bed

Check (✓) Yes or No

PROCEDURE STEPS	Yes	No	COMMENTS
Before, during, and after the procedure, follows Principles-Based Checklist to Use With All Procedures, including: Identifies the patient according to agency policy; attends appropriately to standard precautions, hand hygiene, safety, privacy, and body mechanics.			
1. Obtains the help of a second person to turn patient.			
2. Locks the bed wheels.			
3. Lowers the head of the bed and places patient supine.			
4. Positions self and assistant on opposite sides of the bed.			
5. Lowers the siderails.			
6. Raises the height of the bed to waist level.			
7. Removes the pillow from under patient's head. Places it at the head of the bed.			
8. Ensures that a friction-reducing device, such as a transfer roller sheet, is in place (or places one). Improvises with a plastic bag or film under patient, if needed.			
9. Moves patient to the side of the bed he is turning himself away from by rolling up the drawsheet close to patient's body and pulling.			
10. Aligns patient's legs and head with his trunk.			
11. Places patient's near leg and foot across the far leg (e.g., when turning right, places left leg over right).			
12. Places patient's near arm across his chest. Positions the patient's underneath arm up and away from patient's body.			
13. Stands with a wide base of support with one foot forward of the other.			
14. Grasps drawsheet at level of shoulders and hips.			
15. Places weight on the forward foot.			
16. Bends from the hips and knees.			
17. Instructs patient that the turn will occur on the count of three.			

PROCEDURE STEPS	Yes	No	COMMENTS
18. If positioned on the side toward which patient will turn, flexes own knees and hips and shifts weight to the back foot while pulling on the drawsheet at the hip and shoulder level. If positioned on the opposite side, shifts weight forward.			
19. If a plastic film is used, removes it after turning the patient.			
20. Positions patient's dependent shoulder forward.			
21. Places pillows behind patient's back and between legs to maintain patient in the lateral position.			
22. Replaces the pillow under patient's head.			
23. Places the bed in low position and raises the siderails.			
24. Places the call device within easy reach.			

Recommendation: Pass _____ Needs more practice _____

Student: _____   Date: _____

Instructor: _____   Date: _____

 Copyright © 2016, F. A. Davis Company, Wilkinson & Treas/Procedure Checklists for Fundamentals of Nursing, 3e

PROCEDURE CHECKLIST
Chapter 34: Giving a Back Massage

Check (✓) Yes or No

PROCEDURE STEPS	Yes	No	COMMENTS
Before, during, and after the procedure, follows Principles-Based Checklist to Use With All Procedures, including: Identifies patient according to agency policy using two identifiers; attends appropriately to standard precautions, hand hygiene, safety, privacy, and body mechanics.			
1. Warms the lotion in warm water.			
2. Raises the bed to working height.			
3. Positions patient comfortably on side or prone; keeps siderail raised on opposite side of the bed.			
4. Unties patient's gown and exposes back.			
5. Washes patient's back with warm water if needed.			
6. Puts lotions on own hands.			
7. Places hands on either side of the spine at the base of the neck; using a gentle, continuous pressure, rubs down the length of the spine and then up the sides of the back. Repeats several times.			
8. Does not rub directly over the spine.			
9. Next, applies gentle thumb pressure on either side of the spine at mid-back, pushing outward for about an inch. Repeats from the mid-back to the base of the neck in a series of small, outward strokes.			
10. Always applies pressure away from the spine, not toward it.			
11. Asks patient if the amount of pressure is comfortable.			
12. If unable to massage both sides of the spine at the same time, works on one side and then the other.			
13. Next, moves to the spots that felt the tightest or that patient states are tight, and works in small circles, using gentle thumb pressure.			
14. Using palm of hand, gently shakes one scapula and then the other.			
15. Using horizontal strokes from near the spine across the bottom of the scapula, pushes out all the way across the scapula from the spine. Moves up and repeats until the entire scapula and top of shoulder have been covered.			

PROCEDURE STEPS	Yes	No	COMMENTS
16. If tender spots are located, applies pressure using the fleshy parts of the fingers in a small circular motion.			
17. Begins at the upper shoulder and works down to the lower back, applying pressure in medium-sized circles down each side of the spine with the heels of the hands.			
18. Takes care not to apply too much pressure; assesses patient for comfort.			
19. Next, using horizontal strokes from near the spine below the scapula, pushes out from the spine across to the ribs and works down across the lower back with heels of hands.			
20. With long strokes, gently rubs hands up both sides of the spine from the base of the back to the base of the neck, and then down the sides of the back. Repeats several times.			
21. If unable to do a complete back massage, asks patient where he is most uncomfortable and massages those areas. If patient has general tightness, uses long strokes down each side of the spine and back up the sides.			

Recommendation: Pass _____ Needs more practice _____

Student: _____   Date: _____

Instructor: _____   Date: _____

288   Copyright © 2016, F. A. Davis Company, Wilkinson & Treas/Procedure Checklists for Fundamentals of Nursing, 3e

PROCEDURE CHECKLIST
Chapter 35: Applying Bandages

Check (✔) Yes or No

PROCEDURE STEPS	Yes	No	COMMENTS
Before, during, and after the procedure, follows Principles-Based Checklist to Use With All Procedures, including: Identifies the patient according to agency policy using two identifiers; attends appropriately to standard precautions, hand hygiene, safety, privacy, and body mechanics.			
Before All Bandaging:			
1. Chooses a bandage of the proper width.			
2. Thoroughly cleans and dries the part to be covered. Uses a nontoxic cleansing solution.			
3. Removes excess fluid by gently patting the wound and surrounding skin with gauze sponge.			
4. Works from distal to proximal (peripheral to central).			
5. If a wound is present, applies a primary dressing, as prescribed, over the wound with enough pressure to provide the needed support, but does not bandage too tightly.			
6. Makes sure circulation to the area is not interrupted.			
7. Begins the wrap with the bandage against the skin. Unwinds the bandage as if rolling it over the extremity.			
8. Pads bony prominences before bandaging if there are pressure concerns.			
Circular Turns:			
9. With one hand, holds one end of the bandage in place. With the other hand, encircles the body part two times with the bandage—these first two wraps should completely cover the previous wraps.			
10. Wraps each turn using a 30° angle.			
11. Continues to wrap the body part by overlapping two-thirds the width of the bandage.			
12. Wraps each turn using a 30° angle.			
13. Completes the wrap by making two circular turns.			
14. If circular turns are not being combined with another technique, secures the bandage with tape or metal clips when finished.			

PROCEDURE STEPS	Yes	No	COMMENTS
15. Assesses circulation and comfort of the body part.			
Spiral Turns:			
Follows Steps 1–7, above.			
16. Anchors the bandage by making two circular turns.			
17. Continues to wrap the extremity by encircling the body part with each turn angled at approximately 30°, overlapping the preceding wrap by two-thirds the width of the bandage.			
18. Completes the wrap by making two circular turns and securing the bandage with tape or metal clips.			
Spiral Reverse Turns:			
Follows Steps 1–7, above.			
19. Anchors the bandage by making two circular turns.			
20. Brings the next wrap up at a 30° angle.			
21. Places the thumb of the nondominant hand on the wrap to hold the bandage.			
22. Folds the bandage back on itself, and continues to wrap at a 30° angle in the opposite direction.			
23. Continues to wrap the bandage, overlapping each turn by two-thirds. Aligns each bandage turn at the same position on the extremity.			
24. Completes the wrap by making two circular turns and securing the bandage with tape or metal clips.			
Figure-8 Turns:			
Follows Steps 1–7, above.			
25. Anchors the bandage by making two circular turns.			
26. Wraps the bandage by ascending above the joint and descending below the joint to form a figure 8. Continues to wrap the bandage, overlapping each turn by two-thirds. Aligns each bandage turn at the same position on the extremity.			
27. Completes the wrap by making two circular turns and securing the bandage with tape or metal clips.			
Recurrent Turns:			
Follows Steps 1–10, above.			
28. Anchors the bandage by making two circular turns.			

PROCEDURE STEPS	Yes	No	COMMENTS
29. Folds the bandage back on itself; holds it against the body part with one hand. With the other hand, makes a half turn perpendicular to the circle turns and central to the distal end being bandaged.			
30. Holds the central turn with one hand, and folds the bandage back on itself; brings it over the distal end of the body part to the right of the center, overlapping the center turn by two-thirds the width of the bandage.			
31. Next, holds the bandage at the center with one hand while bringing the bandage back over the end to the left of center. Continues holding and folding the bandage back on itself, alternating right and left until the body part is covered. Overlaps by two-thirds the bandage width with each turn.			
32. Starts and returns each turn to the midline or center of the body part, and angles it slightly more each time to continue covering the body part.			
33. Completes the bandage by making two circular turns and securing the bandage with tape or metal clips.			
After All Bandaging:			
34. After bandaging, assesses circulation and comforts regularly.			

Recommendation: Pass _____ Needs more practice _____

Student: _____   Date: _____

Instructor: _____   Date: _____

Copyright © 2016, F. A. Davis Company, Wilkinson & Treas/Procedure Checklists for Fundamentals of Nursing, 3e

PROCEDURE CHECKLIST
Chapter 35: Applying Binders

Check (✓) Yes or No

PROCEDURE STEPS	Yes	No	COMMENTS
Before, during, and after the procedure, follows Principles-Based Checklist to Use With All Procedures, including: Identifies the patient according to agency policy using two identifiers; attends appropriately to standard precautions, hand hygiene, safety, privacy, and body mechanics.			
1. Chooses a binder of the proper size. Measures.			
2. Washes hands. Dons gloves.			
3. Thoroughly cleans and dries the part to be covered.			
4. Places the body part in its natural, comfortable position (e.g., with the joint slightly flexed) whenever possible.			
5. Pads between skin surfaces (e.g., under the axilla) and over bony prominences.			
6. Fastens from the bottom up.			
7. Changes binders whenever they become soiled or wet.			
Applying an Abdominal Binder:			
8. Measures patient for the abdominal binder. a. Places patient in supine position.			
b. With a disposable measuring tape, encircles the abdomen at the level of the umbilicus. Notes the measurement. This is the length of the binder.			
c. Measures the distance from the costal margin to the top of the iliac crests. This is the width of the binder.			
d. Disposes of gloves and measuring tape, and washes hands.			
e. Based on the measurements, obtains an abdominal binder.			
9. Assists patient to roll to one side. Rolls one end of the binder to the center mark. Places the rolled section of the abdominal binder underneath patient. Positions the binder appropriately between the costal margin and iliac crest.			
10. Makes sure the binder does not slip upward or downward.			
11. Assists patient to turn to the other side while unrolling the binder from underneath him.			

PROCEDURE STEPS	Yes	No	COMMENTS
12. With the dominant hand, grasps the end of the binder on the side farthest from self, and steadily pulls toward the center of patient's abdomen. With the nondominant hand, grasps the end of binder closest to self, and pulls toward the center. Overlaps the ends of the binder so that the Velcro® enclosures meet.			
13. Removes the abdominal binder every 2 hours, and assesses the underlying skin and dressings. Changes wound dressings if they are soiled, or as prescribed.			
Applying a Triangular Arm Binder:			
14. Asks patient to place the affected arm in a natural position across the chest, elbow flexed slightly.			
15. Places one end of the triangle over the shoulder of the uninjured arm, and allows the triangle to fall open so that the elbow of the injured arm is at the apex of the triangle.			
16. Moves the sling behind the injured arm.			
17. Pulls up the lower corner of the triangle over the injured arm to the shoulder of the injured arm.			
18. Ties the sling with a square knot at the neck on the side of the arm requiring support.			
19. Adjusts the injured arm within the sling to ensure patient comfort.			
Applying a T-Binder:			
20. Positions the waist tails under patient at the natural waistline. Brings the right and left tails together, and secures them at the waist with pins or clips.			
21. For a single T-binder, brings the center tail up between patient's legs. Secures the tail at the waist with pins or clips.			
22. For a double T-binder, brings the tails up on either side of the penis. Secures the tail at the waist with pins or clips.			
23. Fastens the ties at the waste using pins or clips.			

Recommendation: Pass _____ Needs more practice _____

Student: _____ Date: _____

Instructor: _____ Date: _____

PROCEDURE CHECKLIST
Chapter 35: Applying a Hydrating Dressing (Hydrocolloid or Hydrogel)

Check (✓) Yes or No

PROCEDURE STEPS	Yes	No	COMMENTS
Before, during, and after the procedure, follows Principles-Based Checklist to Use With All Procedures, including: Identifies the patient according to agency policy using two identifiers; attends appropriately to standard precautions, hand hygiene, safety, privacy, and body mechanics.			
1. Places patient in a comfortable position that provides easy access to the wound.			
2. If a dressing is present, washes hands, applies clean gloves, and removes the old dressing.			
3. Disposes of the soiled dressing and gloves in the biohazard waste receptacle.			
4. Washes hands. Applies clean gloves.			
5. Cleanses the skin surrounding the wound with normal saline or a mild cleansing agent. Rinses the skin well if a cleanser is used.			
6. Allows the skin to dry.			
7. Does not attempt to remove residue that is left on the skin from the old dressing.			
8. Cleanses the wound as directed.			
9. Uses clean or sterile technique, depending on the type of wound.			
10. Assesses the condition of the wound; notes the size, location, type of tissue present, amount of exudate, and odor.			
11. Applies skin prep to the area covered by tape.			
12. Removes soiled gloves; disposes appropriately.			
13. With backing still intact, cuts the hydrocolloid dressing to the desired shape and size. The hydrocolloid dressing should extend 3–4 cm (1.5 in.) beyond the wound margin on all sides.			
14. Applies clean gloves.			
15. Removes the backing of the hydrocolloid dressing, starting at one edge. Places the exposed adhesive portion on patient's skin.			
16. Positions the dressing to provide coverage of the wound.			

PROCEDURE STEPS	Yes	No	COMMENTS
17. Gradually peels away the remaining liner and smooths the hydrocolloid dressing onto the skin by placing a hand on top of the dressing and holding in place for 1 minute.			
18. Assists patient to a comfortable position and removes gloves.			
19. Washes hands.			

Recommendation: Pass _____ Needs more practice _____

Student: _____   Date: _____

Instructor: _____   Date: _____

 Copyright © 2016, F. A. Davis Company, Wilkinson & Treas/Procedure Checklists for Fundamentals of Nursing, 3e

PROCEDURE CHECKLIST

Chapter 35: Applying a Negative Pressure Wound Therapy (NPWT) Device

Check (✓) Yes or No

PROCEDURE STEPS	Yes	No	COMMENTS
Before, during, and after the procedure, follows Principles-Based Checklist to Use With All Procedures, including: Identifies the patient according to agency policy using two identifiers; attends appropriately to standard precautions, hand hygiene, safety, privacy, pain management and body mechanics.			
Removing the Soiled Dressing:			
1. Considers administering pain medication before initiating negative pressure wound therapy. Allows sufficient time for the medication to take effect.			
2. Selects the appropriate dressing (per NPWT system used) to fill the entire wound cavity.			
3. Sets up the prescribed suction pump unit.			
4. Places the waterproof bag or trash receptacle within easy reach during the procedure.			
5. Assists patient to a comfortable position that allows for easy access to the wound.			
6. Positions patient so that gravity will direct the flow of the irrigant from the clean end toward the dirty end of the wound.			
7. Exposes the wound area and drapes patient (uses bath blanket if needed) to expose only the wound area.			
8. Places a waterproof pad as needed.			
9. Prepares a sterile or clean field and adds all supplies: gloves, scissors, irrigation supplies, gauze pad, selected wound dressings, tubing, and/or connectors.			
10. Dons sterile or clean procedure gloves. Uses gown and goggles if exposure to bodily fluids may occur.			
11. Irrigates the wound with 10–30 mL of normal saline or other prescribed solution before all dressing changes.			

PROCEDURE STEPS	Yes	No	COMMENTS
12. Removes the excess solution from the wound. Cleans and dries periwound skin with sterile gauze sponge, as needed. Considers a skin protectant around the wound edges.			
13. Removes soiled gloves and dons new, nonsterile ones for the procedure.			
14. Applies appropriate dressing per preferred NPWT unit.			
Open-Pore Reticulated Polyurethane Foam (i.e., Vacuum-Assisted Closure (V.A.C.) Therapy):			
15. Selects the appropriate foam dressing: black, white, or silver.			
16. Cuts foam dressing to appropriate size to fill the wound cavity. Does not cut the foam dressing over the wound because particles may fall into the wound. Rubs cut edges to remove any loose pieces.			
17. Gently places foam dressing into the cavity without overlapping onto intact skin. Does not overfill the cavity or pack into deep crevices. Does not place foam into blind/unexplored tunnels.			
18. Does not allow foam dressing to overlap onto healthy skin.			
19. If using more than one piece, notes the total number of pieces that were placed into the wound to be documented on the transparent dressing and in patient record.			
20. Applies liquid skin preparation product to periwound, if needed.			
21. Applies transparent film/drape 3–5 cm (1–2 in.) from wound margins without pulling, stretching, or wrinkling the drape. Does not push down or compress foam while placing drape.			
22. Avoids placing dressings all the way around an extremity. If necessary, places several smaller pieces of drape rather than one continuous piece.			
23. Identifies site over the dressing for suction track tubing apparatus.			
24. Pinches up a piece of drape and cuts at least a 2-cm round hole. Does not make a slit or X, as this may close off under pressure.			

PROCEDURE STEPS	Yes	No	COMMENTS
25. Places track adhesive directly over the hole in the drape and applies gentle pressure to secure.			
26. Connects the suction track tubing to the canister tubing and opens clamps.			
27. Turns on power to pump and sets to the prescribed therapy settings to initiate therapy.			
28. Follows Steps 37–43, below.			
Gauze Dressing Application (i.e., Chariker–Jeter Method):			
29. Measures the length of the drain from the wound margin, starting with the first hole perforation and pulls back 1 cm.			
30. Moistens gauze with normal saline.			
31. Wraps or "sandwiches" drain in the moistened gauze and places in wound base. Tucks gauze into any undermining areas to ensure contact with wound bed.			
32. Applies a strip or dollop of ostomy paste 1 cm from the wound edge and secures drain as needed.			
33. Applies liquid skin preparation product to periwound, if needed. Extra drape, hydrocolloid, or transparent dressing may be used to protect fragile skin.			
34. Applies transparent film 1–2 cm (0.5–1 in.) beyond the wound margin to intact skin. Pinches the film around the drain tubing to ensure a tight seal.			
35. Avoids placing circumferential dressings around an extremity. If necessary, places several smaller pieces of drape rather than one continuous piece.			
36. Attaches filter tubing to the canister spout.			
37. Connects tubing from the dressing to the evacuation tubing going to the collection canister.			
38. Positions the tubing and connector away from bony prominences and skin creases.			
39. Ensures clamps are open on all tubing.			
40. Turns on power to pump and sets to the prescribed therapy settings to initiate therapy.			
41. Listens for audible leaks and observes dressing collapse as pressure is applied to the wound bed.			

PROCEDURE STEPS	Yes	No	COMMENTS
42. If the dressing does not collapse or if alarm sounds: a. Presses firmly around the transparent dressing to seal.			
b. Verifies that the machine is turned on, and that all clamps are open and tubing is not kinked.			
c. Checks tubing and drape for leaks. Listens for leaks with a stethoscope or by moving a hand around the wound margins while applying slight pressure.			
d. Does not place multiple layers of drape or adhesive dressing.			
e. Never leaves foam in place without an adequate seal for more than 2 hours. If an adequate seal cannot be achieved in that time, removes the foam and applies a saline-moistened gauze dressing.			
43. Changes the canister at least once a week or when it is filled. Writes the date on the canister.			

Recommendation: Pass _____ Needs more practice _____

Student: _____   Date: _____

Instructor: _____   Date: _____

 Copyright © 2016, F. A. Davis Company, Wilkinson & Treas/Procedure Checklists for Fundamentals of Nursing, 3e

PROCEDURE CHECKLIST
Chapter 35: Applying a Transparent Film Dressing

Check (✓) Yes or No

PROCEDURE STEPS	Yes	No	COMMENTS
Before, during, and after the procedure, follows Principles-Based Checklist to Use With All Procedures, including: Identifies the patient according to agency policy using two identifiers; attends appropriately to standard precautions, hand hygiene, safety, privacy, and body mechanics.			
1. Places patient in a comfortable position that provides easy access to the wound.			
2. If a dressing is present, washes hands, applies clean nonsterile gloves, and removes the old dressing.			
3. Disposes of the soiled dressing and gloves in the biohazard waste receptacle.			
4. Applies clean gloves.			
5. Cleanses the skin surrounding the wound with normal saline or a mild cleansing agent. Rinses the skin well if using a cleanser. Allows the skin to dry.			
6. Applies a skin barrier around the wound before transparent film dressing application.			
7. Removes the center backing liner from the transparent film dressing.			
8. Holding the dressing by the edges, applies the transparent film to the wound without stretching or pulling the dressing or the skin.			
9. Removes the edging liner from the dressing.			
10. Gently smooths and secures the dressing to skin.			
11. Disposes of soiled equipment, and removes gloves.			
12. To remove the dressing: a. Grasps one edge of the film dressing.			
b. Gently lifts the edge.			
c. Stabilizes the skin underneath the elevated edge with a finger.			
d. With the other hand, slowly peels the dressing back over itself, "low and slow," in the direction of hair growth.			

PROCEDURE STEPS	Yes	No	COMMENTS

Recommendation: Pass _____ Needs more practice _____

Student: _____   Date: _____

Instructor: _____   Date: _____

PROCEDURE CHECKLIST
Chapter 35: Emptying a Closed Wound Drainage System

Check (✓) Yes or No

PROCEDURE STEPS	Yes	No	COMMENTS
Before, during, and after the procedure, follows Principles-Based Checklist to Use With All Procedures, including: Identifies the patient according to agency policy using two identifiers; attends appropriately to standard precautions, hand hygiene, safety, privacy, and body mechanics.			
1. Reads the instructions on the drainage device.			
2. Dons procedure gloves, goggles, and mask.			
3. Unpins the drainage device from patient's gown.			
4. Opens the drainage port, and empties the drainage into a small graduated container.			
5. With the port still open, places the collection device on a firm, flat surface.			
6. Uses the palm of one hand to press down on the device and eject air from it. Does not stand directly over the air vent.			
7. Uses the other hand to scrub the port and plug with an alcohol-based antiseptic or povidone-iodine (Betadine) swab, if patient is not allergic to iodine.			
8. Continues to press down on the device and replaces the plug in the port.			
9. Repins the drainage device to patient's gown.			
10. Measures the drainage in the graduated container; discards drainage in the toilet.			
11. Removes gloves.			
12. Records the amount and type of drainage. Reports excess volume to the primary care provider. Notes the date and time on patient's record.			

Recommendation: Pass _____ Needs more practice _____

Student: _____   Date: _____

Instructor: _____   Date: _____

PROCEDURE CHECKLIST
Chapter 35: Obtaining a Wound Culture by Swab

Check (✓) Yes or No

PROCEDURE STEPS	Yes	No	COMMENTS
Before, during, and after the procedure, follows Principles-Based Checklist to Use With All Procedures, including: Identifies the patient according to agency policy using two identifiers; attends appropriately to standard precautions, hand hygiene, safety, privacy, and body mechanics.			
1. Places patient in a comfortable position that provides easy access to the wound and will allow the irrigation solution to flow freely from the wound, with the assistance of gravity.			
2. Places a water-resistant disposable drape and emesis basin to protect the bedding from any runoff.			
3. After washing and drying the hands, applies a clean nonsterile gloves.			
4. Removes the soiled dressing. Disposes of gloves and soiled dressing in a biohazard bag.			
5. Applies clean gloves.			
6. Attaches a 19-gauge angiocatheter to a 35-mL syringe and fills it with normal saline irrigation solution.			
7. Holding the angiocatheter tip 2 cm from the wound bed, gently irrigates the wound with a back-and-forth motion, moving from the superior aspect to the inferior aspect.			
8. Disposes of the syringe and angiocatheter in the sharps container, and gloves in the biohazard waste.			
9. Obtains an aerobic culturette tube and twists the top of the tube to loosen the swab.			
10. Applies clean gloves and locates an area of red, granulating tissue in the wound bed.			
Using Levine Technique:			
11. Withdraws the swab from the aerobic culturette tube. Presses the swab against the granulating area and rotates the swab with sufficient pressure to express fluid from the wound tissue.			

PROCEDURE STEPS	Yes	No	COMMENTS
Using Z-stroke Technique:			
12. Swabs the wound from margin to margin in a 10-point, zigzag pattern, avoiding contact with the wound edge.			
a. Does not allow the swab to touch anything other than the granulating area of the wound.			
b. Does not swab culture areas with slough or eschar present.			
13. Carefully inserts the swab back into the culturette tube, making sure it does not make contact with the opening of tube upon reinsertion.			
14. Twists the cap to secure the tube.			
15. Crushes the ampule of culture medium at the bottom of the tube. (*Note:* Inspects the culture tube used to determine if this step is required.)			
16. Labels the culturette tube with patient's name, patient identifier, birth date, source of specimen, and date and time of collection. (Labels may be provided with the culturette kit.)			
17. Applies a clean dressing to the wound as prescribed.			
18. Arranges for transport of the specimen.			

Recommendation: Pass _____ Needs more practice _____

Student: _____   Date: _____

Instructor: _____   Date: _____

Chapter 35: Performing a Sterile Wound Irrigation

Check (✓) Yes or No

PROCEDURE STEPS	Yes	No	COMMENTS
Before, during, and after the procedure, follows Principles-Based Checklist to Use With All Procedures, including: Identifies the patient according to agency policy using two identifiers; attends appropriately to standard precautions, hand hygiene, safety, privacy, and body mechanics.			
1. Administers pain medication 30 minutes before the procedure, if necessary.			
2. Places patient in a comfortable position that provides easy access to the wound and will allow the irrigation solution to flow freely from the wound, with the assistance of gravity.			
3. Positions a water-resistant disposable drape to protect the bedding from any possible runoff.			
4. After washing and drying hands, applies a gown, face shield, and clean gloves.			
5. Removes the soiled dressing. Disposes of gloves and soiled dressing in a biohazard bag.			
6. Sets up a sterile field on a clean, dry surface.			
7. Adds the following supplies to the field: Sterile gauze Sterile bowl Dressing supplies *Variation A*: A 19-gauge angiocatheter, 35-mL syringe, and sterile emesis basin, or *Variation B*: A sterile commercial irrigation kit			
8. Pours the tepid irrigation solution into the sterile bowl.			
9. Dons sterile gloves.			
10. Irrigates the wound. a. Places the sterile emesis basin at the bottom of the wound to collect irrigation runoff.			
b. *Using an Angiocatheter:* Attaches the 19-gauge angiocatheter to the 35-mL syringe and fills with the irrigation solution, or *Using a Piston-Tip Syringe:* Fills a piston-tip or bulb syringe with irrigation solution.			

PROCEDURE STEPS	Yes	No	COMMENTS
c. Holding the angiocatheter tip or syringe tip 2 cm from the wound bed, gently irrigates the wound with a back-and-forth motion, moving from the superior aspect to the inferior aspect.			
d. Repeats the irrigation until the solution returns clear.			
11. Removes the basin or sterile container from the base of the wound; pats the skin around the wound dry with sterile gauze, beginning at the top of the wound and working downward.			
12. Dresses the wound as prescribed. Uses a waterproof skin protectant around the wound if drainage is heavy.			
13. Disposes of contaminated irrigation fluid in a biohazardous waste receptacle.			
14. Removes soiled drapes from patient area.			
15. Removes gloves, face shield, and gown; disposes of appropriately (they are biohazardous).			
16. Repositions patient to a comfortable position.			
17. Washes hands.			

Recommendation: Pass _____ Needs more practice _____

Student: _____   Date: _____

Instructor: _____   Date: _____

308   Copyright © 2016, F. A. Davis Company, Wilkinson & Treas/Procedure Checklists for Fundamentals of Nursing, 3e

PROCEDURE CHECKLIST
Chapter 35: Placing Skin Closures

Check (✓) Yes or No

PROCEDURE STEPS	Yes	No	COMMENTS
Removing the Soiled Dressing:			
Before, during, and after the procedure, follows Principles-Based Checklist to Use With All Procedures, including: Identifies the patient according to agency policy using two identifiers; attends appropriately to standard precautions, hand hygiene, safety, privacy, and body mechanics.			
1. Dons procedure gloves.			
2. Cleanses the skin at least 5 cm (2 in.) around the wound with saline- or water-moistened gauze. Pats the skin dry, allowing it to dry thoroughly.			
3. Applies skin preparation product, and allows it to dry (or follows agency procedures). Does not allow skin preparation product to come in contact with the wound.			
4. Peels back package tabs to access the adhesive closures.			
5. Removes the card from the package using sterile technique as necessary.			
6. Grasps the end of the skin closure with forceps or gloved hand and peels a strip from the card at a 90° angle.			
7. Starting at the middle of the wound, applies strips across the wound, drawing the wound edges together. Applies closures without tension; does not stretch or strap closures.			
8. Applies one-half of the closure to the wound margin and presses firmly in place.			
9. Using fingers or forceps, ensures skin edges are approximated.			
10. Presses free half firmly on the other side of the wound.			
11. Places the strips so that they extend at least 2–3 cm (¾–1 in.) on either side of the wound to ensure closure.			
12. Places the wound closure strips 3 mm (⅛ in.) apart along the wound.			

PROCEDURE STEPS	Yes	No	COMMENTS
13. If edges are not accurately approximated or tension has been placed on the skin, removes the closure over affected area, peeling each side toward the wound, and reapplies.			

Recommendation: Pass _____ Needs more practice _____

Student: _____ Date: _____

Instructor: _____ Date: _____

PROCEDURE CHECKLIST
Chapter 35: Removing and Applying Dry Dressings

Check (✓) Yes or No

PROCEDURE STEPS	Yes	No	COMMENTS
Before, during, and after the procedure, follows Principles-Based Checklist to Use With All Procedures, including: Identifies the patient according to agency policy using two identifiers; attends appropriately to standard precautions, hand hygiene, safety, privacy, and body mechanics.			
Removing Old Dressing and Cleansing Wound:			
1. Places patient in a comfortable position that provides easy access to the wound.			
2. Washes hands and applies clean procedure gloves.			
3. Loosens the edges of the tape of the old dressing. Stabilizes the skin with one hand while pulling the tape in the opposite direction.			
4. Beginning at the edges of the dressing, lifts the dressing toward the center of the wound.			
5. If the dressing sticks, moistens it with 0.9% (normal) saline before completely removing it.			
6. Assesses the type and amount of drainage present on the soiled dressing.			
7. Disposes of soiled dressing and gloves in a biohazard receptacle.			
8. Removes the cover of a tray of sterile 4 in. × 4 in. gauze. Moistens the gauze with sterile saline.			
9. Applies clean gloves.			
10. Gently cleanses the wound with the saline-moistened gauze by lightly wiping a section of the wound from the center toward the wound edge.			
11. Discards the gauze in a biohazard receptacle and repeats in the next section, using a new piece of gauze with each wiping pass.			
12. Discards gloves and soiled gauze into a biohazard bag.			
13. Reassesses wound for size, color of tissue present, amount and type of exudate, and odor.			

PROCEDURE STEPS	Yes	No	COMMENTS
Applying the Dry Dressing:			
1. Washes hands.			
2. Opens sterile gauze packages on a clean, dry surface.			
3. Applies clean gloves.			
4. Applies a layer of dry dressings over the wound; if drainage is expected, uses an additional layer of dressings.			
5. Places strips of tape at the ends of the dressing and evenly spaced over the remainder of the dressing. Uses strips that are sufficiently long to secure the dressing in place.			
6. Removes gloves, turning them inside out, and discards in a biohazard receptacle.			
7. Assists the patient to a comfortable position.			

Recommendation: Pass _____ Needs more practice _____

Student: _____ Date: _____

Instructor: _____ Date: _____

 Copyright © 2016, F. A. Davis Company, Wilkinson & Treas/Procedure Checklists for Fundamentals of Nursing, 3e

PROCEDURE CHECKLIST
Chapter 35: Removing and Applying Wet-to-Damp Dressings

Check (✓) Yes or No

PROCEDURE STEPS	Yes	No	COMMENTS
Before, during, and after the procedure, follows Principles-Based Checklist to Use With All Procedures, including: Identifies the patient according to agency policy using two identifiers; attends appropriately to standard precautions, hand hygiene, safety, privacy, and body mechanics.			
Removing the Soiled Dressing:			
1. Assesses for pain and medicates 30 minutes before the procedure, if needed.			
2. Places patient in a comfortable position that provides easy access to the wound.			
3. Washes hands and applies clean gloves.			
4. Loosens the edges of the tape of the old dressing. Stabilizes the skin with the other hand, gently raising the edge until taut. Pushes the skin off of the tape in the opposite direction.			
5. Beginning with the top layer, lifts the dressing from the corner toward the center of the wound. If dressing sticks, moistens with 0.9% (normal) saline or tap water before completely removing it.			
6. Continues to remove layers until the entire dressing is removed.			
7. Assesses the type and amount of drainage present on the soiled dressing.			
8. Disposes of soiled dressing and gloves in a biohazard receptacle.			
9. Removes the cover of a tray of sterile 4 in. × 4 in. gauze; moistens the gauze with sterile saline.			
10. Applies clean gloves.			
11. Gently cleanses the wound with the saline-moistened gauze by lightly wiping a section of the wound from the center toward the wound edge.			
12. Assesses the wound for location, amount of tissue present, exudate, and odor.			
13. Discards the gauze in a biohazard receptacle and repeats in the next section using a new piece of gauze with each wiping pass.			
14. Discards gloves and soiled gauze into a biohazard bag. Washes hands.			

PROCEDURE STEPS	Yes	No	COMMENTS
Procedure Steps for Applying Wet-to-Damp Dressing:			
15. Establishes a sterile field, using a sterile impermeable barrier.			
16. Opens sterile gauze packs and a Surgipad onto the sterile field. The amount of gauze used will depend on the size of the wound.			
17. Moistens sterile gauze with a sterile 0.9% saline solution or water for irrigation.			
18. Applies clean procedure gloves.			
19. Squeezes out excess moisture from the gauze before applying.			
20. Applies a single layer of moist fine-mesh gauze to the wound, being careful to place gauze in all depressions or crevices of the wound. Uses sterile forceps or cotton applicator to ensure that deep depressions or sinus tracts are filled with gauze.			
21. Applies a secondary moist layer over the first layer. Repeats this process until the wound is completely filled with moistened sterile gauze.			
22. Does not pack the gauze tightly into the wound.			
23. Does not extend the moist dressing onto the surrounding skin.			
24. Covers the moistened gauze with a Surgipad.			
25. Secures the dressing with tape or Montgomery straps.			
26. Disposes of gloves and sterile field materials in the biohazard waste receptacle.			
27. Assists the patient to a comfortable position.			

Recommendation: Pass _____ Needs more practice _____

Student: _____   Date: _____

Instructor: _____   Date: _____

PROCEDURE CHECKLIST
Chapter 35: Removing Sutures and Staples

Check (✓) Yes or No

PROCEDURE STEPS	Yes	No	COMMENTS
Before, during, and after the procedure, follows Principles-Based Checklist to Use With All Procedures, including: Identifies the patient according to agency policy using two identifiers; attends appropriately to standard precautions, hand hygiene, safety, privacy, and body mechanics.			
Removing Sutures:			
1. Washes hands. Dons gloves.			
2. Obtains a suture removal kit. Assesses staples to ensure none have rotated or turned instead of lying flat along the incision.			
3. Uses the forceps to pick up one end of the suture.			
4. Slides the small scissors around the suture, and cuts near the skin.			
5. With the forceps, gently pulls the suture in the direction of the knotted side to remove it.			
Removing Staples:			
1. Washes hands. Dons gloves.			
2. Positions the staple remover so that the lower jaw is on the bottom.			
3. Places both tips of the lower jaw of the remover under the staple.			
4. Ensures the staple is perpendicular to the plane of the skin. If not, repositions the staple with the tips of the lower jaw.			
5. Lifts slightly on the staple, ensuring that it stays perpendicular to the skin.			
6. Continues to lift slightly while gently squeezing the handles together to close.			
7. Lifts the reformed staple straight up from the skin.			
8. Removes every other staple, and checks the tension on the wound.			
9. If there is no significant pull on the wound, removes the remaining staples.			
10. Places the removed staples on a piece of gauze.			
11. Applies dressing if needed.			
12. Disposes of the removed staples in the sharps container.			
13. Removes gloves and washes hands.			

PROCEDURE STEPS	Yes	No	COMMENTS

Recommendation: Pass _____ Needs more practice _____

Student: _____   Date: _____

Instructor: _____   Date: _____

PROCEDURE CHECKLIST
Chapter 35: Shortening a Wound Drain

Check (✓) Yes or No

PROCEDURE STEPS	Yes	No	COMMENTS
Before, during, and after the procedure, follows Principles-Based Checklist to Use With All Procedures, including: Identifies the patient according to agency policy using two identifiers; attends appropriately to standard precautions, hand hygiene, safety, privacy, and body mechanics.			
1. Dons procedure gloves.			
2. Removes wound dressing.			
3. Removes soiled gloves and discards in a moisture-proof, biohazard collection container.			
4. Uses sterile scissors to cut halfway through a sterile gauze dressing (for later use), or uses a sterile precut drain dressing.			
5. If the drain is sutured in place, uses sterile scissors to cut the suture.			
6. Firmly grasps the full width of the drain at the level of the skin and pulls it out by the prescribed amount (e.g., 6 mm [¼ in.]).			
7. Inserts a sterile safety pin through the drain at the level of the skin. Holds the drain tightly, and inserts the pin above own fingers.			
8. Using sterile scissors, cuts off the drain at about 2.5 cm (1 in.) above the skin.			
9. Cleanses the wound, using sterile gauze swabs and the prescribed cleaning solution.			
10. Applies precut sterile gauze around the drain; then redresses the wound.			
11. Removes gloves and discards in a biohazard container.			
12. Leaves patient in a safe and comfortable position.			

Recommendation: Pass _____ Needs more practice _____

Student: _____   Date: _____

Instructor: _____   Date: _____

PROCEDURE CHECKLIST
Chapter 35: Taping a Dressing

Check (✓) Yes or No

PROCEDURE STEPS	Yes	No	COMMENTS
Before, during, and after the procedure, follows Principles-Based Checklist to Use With All Procedures, including: Identifies the patient according to agency policy using two identifiers; attends appropriately to standard precautions, hand hygiene, safety, privacy, and body mechanics.			
1. Washes hands. Dons gloves.			
2. Chooses the type of tape based on wound size, location, amount of drainage or edema, frequency of dressing changes, patient's activity level, and type of dressings used.			
3. Chooses tape of the width that is appropriate for the size of the dressing. The larger the dressing, the wider the tape needed for securing.			
4. Chooses a tape that stretches if the area is at risk for distention, edema, hematoma formation, or movement.			
5. Tears strips that extend ½ inch beyond the dressing.			
6. Places tape perpendicular to the incision.			
7. When taping over joints, applies the tape at a right angle to the direction of joint movement, or at a right angle to a body crease. For example, tapes a shoulder or knee horizontally, not lengthwise.			
8. Applies tape without tension or pulling.			
9. Smooths tape in place by gently stroking the surface to maximize adhesion.			
10. Replaces tape if site becomes edematous, or skin is not intact.			

Recommendation: Pass _____ Needs more practice _____

Student: _____   Date: _____

Instructor: _____   Date: _____

Copyright © 2016, F. A. Davis Company, Wilkinson & Treas/Procedure Checklists for Fundamentals of Nursing, 3e

Chapter 36: Administering Oxygen (by Cannula, Face Mask, or Face Tent)

Check (✓) Yes or No

PROCEDURE STEPS	Yes	No	COMMENTS
Before, during, and after the procedure, follows Principles-Based Checklist to Use With All Procedures, including: Identifies the patient according to agency policy using two identifiers; attends appropriately to standard precautions, hand hygiene, safety, privacy, body mechanics, and documentation.			
1. Attaches the flow meter to the wall oxygen source. If using a portable oxygen tank, attaches the flow meter to the tank if it is not already connected.			
2. Assembles the oxygen equipment.			
3. Attaches the humidifier to the flow meter. (Humidification is necessary only for flow rates of greater than 3 L/min.) If a humidifier is not used, attaches the adapter to the flow meter.			
4. Turns on the oxygen using the flow meter and adjusts it according to the prescribed flow rate.			
Variation: Nasal Cannula			
5. Attaches the nasal cannula to the humidifier or the adapter.			
6. Places the nasal prongs in patient's nares, then places the tubing around each ear.			
7. Uses the slide adjustment device to tighten the cannula under patient's chin.			
8. Makes sure that the oxygen equipment is set up correctly and functioning properly before leaving patient's bedside.			
9. Assesses respiratory status before leaving bedside.			
Variation: Face Mask			
10. Gently places the face mask on patient's face, applying it from the bridge of the nose to under the chin.			
11. Secures the elastic band around the back of patient's head, making sure the mask fits snugly but comfortably.			
12. Makes sure that the oxygen equipment is set up correctly and functioning properly before leaving patient's bedside.			
13. Assesses respiratory status before leaving bedside.			

PROCEDURE STEPS	Yes	No	COMMENTS
Variation: Face Tent			
14. Gently places the face tent in front of patient's face, making sure that it fits under the chin.			
15. Secures the elastic band around the back of patient's head.			
16. Makes sure that the oxygen equipment is set up correctly and functioning properly before leaving patient's bedside.			
17. Assesses respiratory status before leaving the bedside.			

Recommendation: Pass _____ Needs more practice _____

Student: _____ Date: _____

Instructor: _____ Date: _____

PROCEDURE CHECKLIST
Chapter 36: Caring for Patients Requiring Mechanical Ventilation

Check (✓) Yes or No

PROCEDURE STEPS	Yes	No	COMMENTS
Before, during, and after the procedure, follows Principles-Based Checklist to Use With All Procedures, including: Identifies the patient according to agency policy using two identifiers; attends appropriately to standard precautions, hand hygiene, safety, privacy, body mechanics, and documentation.			
Initial Ventilator Setup:			
1. Prepares a resuscitation bag: Attaches a flow meter to oxygen source; attaches an adapter to the flow meter; and connects the oxygen tubing to the adapter.			
2. Turns on the oxygen and adjusts the flow rate.			
3. The respiratory therapy department is responsible for setting up mechanical ventilators in most agencies. If necessary to perform the setup, refers to the manufacturer's instructions.			
4. Plugs the ventilator into an electrical outlet and turns it on.			
5. Verifies ventilator settings and adjusts them with the prescriber's order.			
6. Checks the ventilator alarm limits. Makes sure they are set appropriately.			
7. Makes sure the humidifier is filled with sterile distilled water.			
8. Dons gloves, gown, and eye protection if has not already done so.			
9. Attaches the ventilator tubing to the endotracheal or tracheostomy tube.			
10. Places the ventilator tubing in the securing device.			
11. Attaches a capnography device, if available.			
12. Prepares the inline (closed) suction equipment. (See Procedure Checklist Chapter 36: Performing Tracheostomy or Endotracheal Suctioning [Inline Closed System].)			
After Initial Ventilator Setup:			
13. Checks ABGs and performs respiratory assessment initially, and again in 30 minutes. Checks ABGs when there are changes in ventilator settings and as patient condition indicates.			

PROCEDURE STEPS	Yes	No	COMMENTS
14. Checks the ventilator tubing frequently for condensation.			
15. Drains the fluid into a collection device or briefly disconnects patient from the ventilator and empties the tubing into a waste receptacle, according to agency policy.			
16. Never drains the fluid into the humidifier.			
17. Keeps the head of the bed elevated 30°–45°.			
18. Checks ventilator and humidifier settings regularly.			
19. Checks the inline thermometer.			
20. Provides an alternative form of communication, such as a letter board or white board.			
21. Repositions regularly (every 1–2 hours), being careful not to pull on the ventilator tubing.			
22. Provides frequent oral care; moistens the lips with a cool, damp cloth and water-based lubricant.			
23. Provides regular antiseptic oral care according to agency policy. One recommended regimen is: a. Brush teeth twice a day with a soft toothbrush.			
b. Moisturize oral mucosa and lips every 2–4 hours.			
c. Use a chlorhexidine gluconate (0.12%) rinse twice a day in adult patients having cardiac surgery.			
d. Use mouthwash twice daily for all adult patients.			
24. Ensures that the call light is always within reach and answers call light and ventilator alarms promptly.			
25. Monitors the tracheostomy tube (if cuffed) for proper cuff inflation (see Clinical Insight 36-4, in Volume 2 of the textbook).			
26. Checks for gastric distention and takes measures to prevent aspiration.			
27. Cleans, disinfects, or changes ventilator tubing and equipment according to agency policy.			

 Copyright © 2016, F. A. Davis Company, Wilkinson & Treas/Procedure Checklists for Fundamentals of Nursing, 3e

PROCEDURE STEPS	Yes	No	COMMENTS
28. Gives sedatives or anti-anxiety agents as needed.			

Recommendation: Pass _____ Needs more practice _____

Student: _____   Date: _____

Instructor: _____   Date: _____

PROCEDURE CHECKLIST
Chapter 36: Inserting a Nasopharyngeal Airway

Check (✓) Yes or No

PROCEDURE STEPS	Yes	No	COMMENTS
Before, during, and after the procedure, follows Principles-Based Checklist to Use With All Procedures, including: Identifies the patient according to agency policy using two identifiers; attends appropriately to standard precautions, hand hygiene, safety, privacy, body mechanics, and documentation.			
1. Performs hand hygiene and dons procedure gloves.			
2. Places patient supine or in semi-Fowler's position.			
3. Explains the procedure to patient.			
4. Validates airway size. Measures airway from tip of nose to jawline below the ear, and uses an airway about 2.5 cm (1 in.) longer than that. Airway should be slightly smaller than the nares.			
5. Lubricates the airway with a water-soluble lubricant.			
6. Tilts patient's head back to hyperextend the neck.			
7. Pushes up the tip of the nose and inserts the tip of airway into the naris.			
8. Advances the airway along the floor of the nostril into the posterior pharynx behind the tongue, until the outer flange rests on the nostril. a. If resistance is met, rotates the tube slightly.			
b. Does not force against resistance.			
9. Asks patient to open his mouth. Depresses the tongue with a tongue blade and inspects the pharynx for proper placement of the tube tip. Uses a penlight, if necessary, for better visualization.			
10. Closes patient's mouth, and places finger close to the tube's opening to feel for air exchange.			
11. Auscultates the lungs for presence of bilateral breath sounds.			
12. Removes the airway at least every 8 hours to check nasal mucosa; cleans airway at that time.			

Recommendation: Pass _____ Needs more practice _____

Student: _____   Date: _____

Instructor: _____   Date: _____

PROCEDURE CHECKLIST
Chapter 36: Inserting an Oropharyngeal Airway

Check (✔) Yes or No

PROCEDURE STEPS	Yes	No	COMMENTS
Before, during, and after the procedure, follows Principles-Based Checklist to Use With All Procedures, including: Identifies the patient according to agency policy using two identifiers; attends appropriately to standard precautions, hand hygiene, safety, privacy, body mechanics, and documentation.			
1. Chooses correct airway size. Length of airway should extend from the front teeth to the end of the jaw line.			
2. Performs hand hygiene and dons procedure gloves.			
3. Explains the procedure to patient.			
4. Clears the mouth of debris or secretions. Suctions prn.			
5. Places patient supine or in semi-Fowler's position with the neck hyperextended.			
6. Gently opens patient's mouth. Removes dentures, if present.			
7. Uses a tongue blade (or crossed fingers technique) to depress the tongue, as needed.			
8. Inserts the airway in the upside-down position (inner curve of the C faces upward toward the nose).			
9. As the airway approaches the posterior wall of the pharynx, rotates it 180°.			
10. Continues inserting until front flange is flush with the lips.			
11. Keeps the head tilted slightly back and the chin elevated.			
12. Does not tape airway in place.			
13. Positions patient on her side.			
14. Provides oral hygiene and cleanses the airway every 2–4 hours.			

Recommendation: Pass _____ Needs more practice _____

Student: _____ Date: _____

Instructor: _____ Date: _____

Copyright © 2016, F. A. Davis Company, Wilkinson & Treas/Procedure Checklists for Fundamentals of Nursing, 3e

PROCEDURE CHECKLIST
Chapter 36: Monitoring Pulse Oximetry (Arterial Oxygen Saturation)

Check (✓) Yes or No

PROCEDURE STEPS	Yes	No	COMMENTS
Before, during, and after the procedure, follows Principles-Based Checklist to Use With All Procedures, including: Identifies the patient according to agency policy using two identifiers; attends appropriately to standard precautions, hand hygiene, safety, privacy, body mechanics, and documentation.			
1. Chooses a sensor appropriate for patient's age, size, and weight; and the desired location.			
2. If patient is allergic to adhesive, uses a clip-on probe sensor. Uses a nasal sensor if patient's peripheral circulation is compromised.			
3. Prepares the site by cleansing and drying.			
4. If the finger is the desired monitoring location, removes nail polish or an acrylic nail, if present.			
5. Removes the protective backing if using a disposable probe sensor that contains adhesive.			
6. Attaches the probe sensor to the chosen site. Makes sure that the photodetector diodes and LED on the probe sensor face each other.			
7. If a clip-on probe sensor is used, warns patient that he may feel a pinching sensation.			
8. Connects the sensor probe to the oximeter and turns it on. Makes sure the oximeter is plugged into an electrical socket.			
9. Checks the pulse rate displayed on the oximeter to see if it correlates with patient's radial pulse.			
10. Reads the SaO_2 measurement on the digital display when it reaches a constant value, usually in 10–30 seconds.			
11. Sets and turns on the alarm limits for SaO_2 and pulse rate, according to the manufacturer's instructions, patient condition, and agency policy, if continuous monitoring is necessary.			
12. Obtains readings as ordered or indicated by patient's respiratory status.			

PROCEDURE STEPS	Yes	No	COMMENTS
13. Rotates the probe site every 4 hours for an adhesive probe sensor and every 2 hours for a clip-on probe sensor, if continuous monitoring is indicated.			
14. Removes the probe sensor and turns off the oximeter when monitoring is no longer necessary.			

Recommendation: Pass _____ Needs more practice _____

Student: _____   Date: _____

Instructor: _____   Date: _____

PROCEDURE CHECKLIST

Chapter 36: Collecting an Expectorated Sputum Specimen

Check (✓) Yes or No

PROCEDURE STEPS	Yes	No	COMMENTS
Before, during, and after the procedure, follows Principles-Based Checklist to Use With All Procedures, including: Identifies the patient according to agency policy using two identifiers; attends appropriately to standard precautions, hand hygiene, safety, privacy, body mechanics, and documentation.			
1. Verifies the medical prescription for type of sputum analysis.			
2. Positions patient in a high or semi-Fowler's position, or sitting on the edge of the bed.			
3. Drapes a towel or linen-saver pad over patient's chest.			
4. Hands patient a glass of water and an emesis basin, and has him gargle and rinse his mouth.			
5. If patient has an abdominal or chest incision, has patient splint the incision with a pillow when coughing.			
6. Provides patient with the specimen container. Advises patient to avoid touching the inside of the container.			
7. If necessary to hold the container for the patient, first dons procedure gloves.			
8. Asks patient to breathe deeply for three or four breaths, and then asks him, after a full inhalation, to hold his breath and then cough.			
9. Instructs patient to expectorate the secretions directly into the specimen container.			
10. Instructs patient to repeat deep breathing and coughing until an adequate sample is obtained.			
11. Dons procedure gloves, if not already wearing them.			
12. Covers the specimen container with the lid immediately after the specimen is collected.			
13. Labels the specimen container with patient identification, the name of the test, and collection date and time.			

PROCEDURE STEPS	Yes	No	COMMENTS
14. Places the specimen in a plastic bag with a biohazard label. Attaches a completed laboratory requisition form.			
15. Sends the specimen immediately to the laboratory, or refrigerates it if transport might be delayed.			

Recommendation: Pass _____ Needs more practice _____

Student: _____   Date: _____

Instructor: _____   Date: _____

PROCEDURE CHECKLIST
Chapter 36: Collecting a Suctioned Sputum Specimen

Check (✓) Yes or No

PROCEDURE STEPS	Yes	No	COMMENTS
Before, during, and after the procedure, follows Principles-Based Checklist to Use With All Procedures, including: Identifies the patient according to agency policy using two identifiers; attends appropriately to standard precautions, hand hygiene, safety, privacy, body mechanics, and documentation.			
1. Positions patient in a high- or semi-Fowler's position.			
2. Drapes a towel or linen-saver pad over patient's chest.			
3. If patient has an abdominal or chest incision, has patient splint the incision with a pillow.			
4. Administers oxygen to patient, if indicated.			
5. Prepares the suction device and makes sure it is functioning properly.			
6. Dons protective eyewear (and gown, if needed).			
7. Attaches the suction tubing to the male adapter of the inline sputum specimen container.			
8. Dons sterile gloves.			
9. Attaches the sterile suction catheter to the flexible tubing of the sputum specimen container. Remembers that the hand that touched the container is no longer sterile. Keeps the dominant hand sterile.			
10. Lubricates the suction catheter with sterile saline solution.			
11. Inserts the tip of the suction catheter gently through the nasopharynx, endotracheal tube, or tracheostomy tube and advances it into the trachea. (See Procedure Checklist Chapter 36: Tracheostomy Care Using Sterile Technique, or Procedure Checklist Chapter 36: Performing Upper Airway Suctioning.)			
12. When patient begins coughing, applies suction for 5–10 seconds to collect the specimen.			
13. If an adequate specimen (5–10 mL) is not obtained, allows patient to rest for 1–2 minutes and then repeats the procedure. Administers oxygen to patient at this time, if indicated.			

PROCEDURE STEPS	Yes	No	COMMENTS
14. When an adequate specimen is collected, discontinues suction, then gently removes the suction catheter.			
15. Removes the suction catheter from the specimen container and disposes of the catheter in the appropriate container.			
16. Removes the suction tubing from the specimen container and connects the flexible tubing on the specimen container to the plastic adapter to close the container.			
17. If sputum comes in contact with the outside of the specimen container, cleans it with a disinfectant according to agency policy.			
18. Offers tissues and provides mouth care.			
19. Labels the specimen container with patient identification, the name of the test, and collection date and time.			
20. Places the specimen in a plastic bag with a biohazard label. Attaches a completed laboratory requisition form.			
21. Sends the specimen to the laboratory immediately or refrigerates it if transport might be delayed.			

Recommendation: Pass _____ Needs more practice _____

Student: _____   Date: _____

Instructor: _____   Date: _____

 Copyright © 2016, F. A. Davis Company, Wilkinson & Treas/Procedure Checklists for Fundamentals of Nursing, 3e

PROCEDURE CHECKLIST
Chapter 36: Performing Nasotracheal Suctioning (Open System)

Check (✓) Yes or No

PROCEDURE STEPS	Yes	No	COMMENTS
Before, during, and after the procedure, follows Principles-Based Checklist to Use With All Procedures, including: Identifies the patient according to agency policy using two identifiers; attends appropriately to standard precautions, hand hygiene, safety, privacy, body mechanics, and documentation.			
1. Positions patient in a semi-Fowler's position with his neck hyperextended (unless contraindicated).			
2. Places the linen-saver pad or towel on patient's chest.			
3. Puts on a face shield or goggles and gown.			
4. Turns on the wall suction or portable suction machine and adjusts the pressure regulator according to agency policy (typically 100–150 mm Hg for adults, 100–120 mm Hg for children, 80–100 for infants, and 60–80 mm Hg for neonates).			
5. Dons a procedure glove and tests the suction equipment by occluding the connection tubing. Then discards glove and performs hand hygiene.			
6. Opens the suction catheter kit or the gathered equipment if a kit isn't available. Opens the water-soluble lubricant and preferably a nasopharyngleal airway (if available).			
7. Dons sterile gloves (alternatively, puts a sterile glove on the dominant hand and a clean procedure glove on the nondominant hand); considers the dominant hand sterile and the nondominant hand nonsterile. If considering both hands sterile, removes cap from sterile water before donning gloves.			
8. Pours sterile saline into the sterile container using the nondominant hand.			
9. Picks up the suction catheter with the dominant hand and attaches it to the connection tubing, maintaining sterility of the hand and the catheter.			

Copyright © 2016, F. A. Davis Company, Wilkinson & Treas/Procedure Checklists for Fundamentals of Nursing, 3e

PROCEDURE STEPS	Yes	No	COMMENTS
10. Puts the tip of the suction catheter into the sterile container of normal saline solution and suctions a small amount of normal saline solution through the suction catheter. Applies suction by placing a finger over the suction control port of the suction catheter.			
11. Asks patient to take several slow deep breaths. If patient's oxygen saturation is less than 94%, or if he is in any distress, may need to give supplemental oxygen before, during, and after suctioning. See Procedure Checklist Chapter 36: Administering Oxygen (by Cannula, Face Mask, or Face Tent).			
12. Using the nondominant hand, removes the oxygen delivery device, if present. If patient is receiving nasal oxygen, places the nasal cannula in patient's mouth.			
13. Premeasures the depth to insert the suction catheter (measures distance between the edge of the mouth to the tip of the earlobe and down to the bottom of the neck [for adults about 20 cm, or 8 in.]); is careful not to contaminate the catheter while measuring.			
14. Lubricates the suction catheter tip with a water-soluble lubricant.			
15. Using the dominant hand, gently but quickly inserts the suction catheter into the naris, through the nasotracheal tube, and down to the pharynx.			
16. Advances the suction catheter with inspiration to the predetermined distance, being careful not to force the catheter.			
17. Places a finger (thumb) over the suction control port of the catheter. Applies suction while withdrawing the catheter, using a continuous rotating motion.			
18. Applies suction for no longer than 15 seconds.			
19. After withdrawing the catheter, clears it by placing the tip of the catheter into the container of sterile saline and applying suction.			
20. Lubricates the catheter and repeats suctioning as needed, allowing intervals of at least 30 seconds between suctioning. Reapplies oxygen between suctioning efforts, if required.			
21. Replaces the oxygen source, as needed.			

338 Copyright © 2016, F. A. Davis Company, Wilkinson & Treas/Procedure Checklists for Fundamentals of Nursing, 3e

PROCEDURE STEPS	Yes	No	COMMENTS
22. Coils the suction catheter in the dominant hand (alternatively, wraps it around the dominant hand). Holds the catheter while pulling the sterile glove off over it. Discards the glove containing the catheter in a biohazard receptacle (e.g., bag) designated by the agency.			
23. Using the nondominant hand, clears the connecting tubing of secretions by placing the tip into the container of sterile saline.			
24. Disposes of equipment and makes sure new suction supplies are readily available for future suctioning.			
25. Provides mouth care.			
26. Positions patient for comfort and allows him to rest.			

Recommendation: Pass _____ Needs more practice _____

Student: _____ Date: _____

Instructor: _____ Date: _____

Check (✓) Yes or No

PROCEDURE STEPS	Yes	No	COMMENTS
Before, during, and after the procedure, follows Principles-Based Checklist to Use With All Procedures, including: Identifies the patient according to agency policy using two identifiers; attends appropriately to standard precautions, hand hygiene, safety, privacy, body mechanics, and documentation.			
1. Positions patient in a semi-Fowler's position with his head turned facing the nurse.			
2. Places the linen-saver pad or towel on patient's chest.			
3. Puts on a face shield or goggles and gown.			
4. Turns on the wall suction or portable suction machine and adjusts the pressure regulator according to agency policy (typically 100–150 mm Hg for adults, 100–120 mm Hg for children, 80–100 mm Hg for infants, and 60–80 mm Hg for neonates).			
5. Dons a procedure glove and tests the suction equipment by occluding the connection tubing. Then discards the glove and performs hand hygiene.			
6. Opens the suction catheter kit or the gathered equipment if a kit isn't available.			
7. Dons sterile gloves (alternatively, puts a sterile glove on the dominant hand and a clean procedure glove on the nondominant hand); considers the dominant hand sterile and the nondominant hand nonsterile. (Note: If both hands are considered sterile, removes the cap from the sterile water before donning gloves.)			
8. Pours sterile saline into the sterile container using the nondominant hand.			
9. Picks up the suction catheter with the dominant hand and attaches it to the connection tubing, maintaining sterility of the hand and the catheter.			
10. Puts the tip of the suction catheter into the sterile container of normal saline solution and suctions a small amount of normal saline solution through the suction catheter. Applies suction by placing a finger over the suction control port of the suction catheter.			

PROCEDURE STEPS	Yes	No	COMMENTS
11. Asks patient to take several slow deep breaths. If patient's oxygen saturation is less than 94%, or if he is in any distress, may need to give supplemental oxygen before, during, and after suctioning. See Procedure Checklist Chapter 36: Administering Oxygen (by Cannula, Face Mask, or Face Tent).			
12. Using the nondominant hand, removes the oxygen delivery device, if present. (If patient is receiving nasal oxygen, does not need to remove it.)			
13. Premeasures the depth to insert the suction catheter (measures distance between the edge of the mouth to the tip of the earlobe and down to the bottom of the neck [for adults about 15 cm, or 6 in.]); is careful not to contaminate the catheter while measuring.			
14. Lubricates the suction catheter tip with normal saline.			
15. Using the dominant hand, gently but quickly inserts the suction catheter along the side of patient's mouth or through the endotracheal tube into the oropharynx.			
16. Advances the suction catheter with inspiration to the predetermined distance, being careful not to force the catheter.			
17. Places a finger (thumb) over the suction control port of the catheter. Applies suction while withdrawing the catheter, using a continuous rotating motion.			
18. Applies suction for no longer than 15 seconds.			
19. After withdrawing the catheter, clears it by placing the tip of the catheter into the container of sterile saline and applying suction.			
20. Lubricates the catheter and repeats suctioning as needed, allowing intervals of at least 30 seconds between suctioning. Reapplies oxygen between suctioning efforts, if required.			
21. Replaces the oxygen source.			
22. Coils the suction catheter in the dominant hand (alternatively, wraps it around the dominant hand). Holds the catheter while pulling the sterile glove off over it. Discards the glove containing the catheter in a biohazard receptacle (e.g., bag) designated by the agency.			

 Copyright © 2016, F. A. Davis Company, Wilkinson & Treas/Procedure Checklists for Fundamentals of Nursing, 3e

PROCEDURE STEPS	Yes	No	COMMENTS
23. Using the nondominant hand, clears the connecting tubing of secretions by placing the tip into the container of sterile saline.			
24. Disposes of equipment and makes sure new suction supplies are readily available for future suctioning.			
25. Provides mouth care.			
26. Positions patient for comfort and allows him to rest.			

Recommendation: Pass _____ Needs more practice _____

Student: _____   Date: _____

Instructor: _____   Date: _____

PROCEDURE CHECKLIST
Chapter 36: Performing Percussion, Vibration, and Postural Drainage

Check (✓) Yes or No

PROCEDURE STEPS	Yes	No	COMMENTS
Before, during, and after the procedure, follows Principles-Based Checklist to Use With All Procedures, including: Identifies the patient according to agency policy using two identifiers; attends appropriately to standard precautions, hand hygiene, safety, privacy, body mechanics, and documentation.			
1. Helps patient assume the appropriate position based on the lung field that requires drainage: a. *Apical areas of the upper lobes*: Asks patient to sit at the edge of the bed. Places a pillow at the base of the spine for support, if needed. If patient is unable to sit at edge of the bed, places him in high Fowler's position.			
b. *Posterior section of the upper lobes*: Positions patient supine with pillow under his hips and knees flexed. Asks patient to rotate slightly away from the side that requires drainage.			
c. *Middle or lower lobes*: Places the bed in Trendelenburg position. Places patient in Sims' position. To drain the left lung, positions patient on his right side. For the right lung, positions patient on his left side.			
d. *Posterior lower lobes*: Keeping the bed flat, positions patient prone with a pillow under his stomach.			
2. Asks patient to remain in the desired position for 10–15 minutes.			
3. Performs percussion over the affected lung area while patient is in the desired drainage position: a. Promotes relaxation by instructing patient to breathe deeply and slowly.			
b. Covers the area to be percussed with a towel or patient's gown.			
c. Avoids clapping over bony prominences, female breasts, or tender areas.			
d. Cups the hands, with fingers flexed and thumbs pressed against the index fingers.			

PROCEDURE STEPS	Yes	No	COMMENTS
e. Places cupped hands over the lung area requiring drainage; percusses the area for 1–3 minutes by alternately striking cupped hands rhythmically against patient.			
4. Performs vibrations while patient remains in the desired drainage position: a. Places the flat surface of one hand over the lung area that requires vibration; places the other hand on top of that hand at a right angle.			
b. Instructs patient to inhale slowly and deeply.			
c. Instructs patient to make an "fff" or "sss" sound as he exhales.			
d. As patient exhales, presses the fingers and palms firmly against patient's chest wall and gently vibrates with the hands over the lung area.			
e. Continues performing vibrations for three exhalations.			
5. After performing postural drainage, percussion, and vibration, allows patient to sit up. Instructs him to cough at the end of a deep inspiration. Suctions patient if he is unable to expectorate secretions.			
6. If a sputum specimen is needed, collects it in a specimen container.			
7. Repeats Steps 1 through 5 for each lung field that requires treatment.			
8. The entire treatment does not exceed 60 minutes.			
9. Provides mouth care.			

Recommendation: Pass _____ Needs more practice _____

Student: _____   Date: _____

Instructor: _____   Date: _____

PROCEDURE CHECKLIST
Chapter 36: Performing Tracheostomy or Endotracheal Suctioning (Open System)

Check (✓) Yes or No

PROCEDURE STEPS	Yes	No	COMMENTS
Before, during, and after the procedure, follows Principles-Based Checklist to Use With All Procedures, including: Identifies the patient according to agency policy using two identifiers; attends appropriately to standard precautions, hand hygiene, safety, privacy, body mechanics, and documentation.			
Note: This procedure uses modified sterile technique.			
1. Positions patient in a semi-Fowler's position, unless contraindicated.			
2. Places a linen-saver pad or towel on patient's chest.			
3. Turns on the wall suction or portable suction machine and adjusts the pressure regulator according to agency policy (typically 100–150 mm Hg for adults, 100–120 mm Hg for children, and 50–95 mm Hg for infants).			
4. Dons a nonsterile glove and face shield or goggles.			
5. Tests the suction equipment by occluding the connection tubing.			
6. Removes and discards the glove and performs hand hygiene.			
7. Opens the suction catheter kit or the gathered supplies if a kit is not available.			
8. Pours sterile saline into the sterile container, using the nondominant hand.			
9. Dons sterile gloves. Considers the dominant hand sterile and the nondominant hand nonsterile. (Some guidelines allow for clean procedure gloves; follow agency policy.)			
10. Premeasures the catheter insertion distance for 0.5 to 1 cm (¼ to ½ in.) past the distal end of the endotracheal tube (ETT); the ETT normally sits between 3 and 7 cm (1 to 2¾ in.) above the carina.			
11. Picks up the suction catheter with the dominant hand and attaches it to the connection tubing. Keeps dominant hand sterile (clean).			

PROCEDURE STEPS	Yes	No	COMMENTS
12. Puts the tip of the suction catheter into the sterile container of normal saline solution and suctions a small amount of normal saline solution through the catheter. Applies suction by placing a finger over the suction control port of the suction catheter.			
13. If patient is receiving oxygen, hyperoxygenates according to agency policy: a. *Patient requiring mechanical ventilation*: Presses the 100% O_2 button on the ventilator or attaches the resuscitation bag to the endotracheal tube or tracheostomy tube and manually hyperoxygenates patient according to agency policy. Removes the resuscitation bag and places it next to patient when finished.			
b. *Patient not requiring mechanical ventilation*: Obtains help from an assistant. Asks the assistant to attach the resuscitation bag to the tracheostomy or endotracheal tube. Hyperoxygenates patient by compressing the resuscitation bag three to five times. Removes the resuscitation bag and places it next to patient when finished.			
14. Lubricates the suction catheter tip with normal saline.			
15. Using the dominant hand, gently but quickly inserts the suction catheter into the endotracheal tube or tracheostomy tube.			
16. Advances the suction catheter, with suction off, gently aiming downward and being careful not to force the catheter. Inserts to the premeasured length, not more than 15 cm (6 in.).			
17. Applies suction while withdrawing the catheter. Rotates catheter while withdrawing.			
18. Does not apply suction for longer than 15 seconds.			
19. Repeats suctioning as needed, allowing at least 30-second intervals between suctioning.			
20. Hyperoxygenates patient between each pass.			
21. Limits total suctioning time to 5 minutes.			
22. Replaces the oxygen source, if patient was removed from the source during suctioning.			
23. Coils the suction catheter in the dominant hand (alternatively, wraps it around the dominant hand). Pulls the sterile glove off over the coiled catheter.			
24. Discards the glove and catheter in a water-resistant receptacle designated by the agency.			
25. Dons clean procedure gloves and provides mouth care.			

PROCEDURE STEPS	Yes	No	COMMENTS
26. Using the nondominant hand, clears the connecting tubing of secretions by placing the tip into the container of sterile saline.			
27. Turns off the oxygen and suction units.			
28. Repositions patient, as needed.			

Recommendation: Pass _____ Needs more practice _____

Student: _____ Date: _____

Instructor: _____ Date: _____

Chapter 36: Performing Tracheostomy or Endotracheal Suctioning
(Inline Closed System)

Check (✓) Yes or No

PROCEDURE STEPS	Yes	No	COMMENTS
Before, during, and after the procedure, follows Principles-Based Checklist to Use With All Procedures, including: Identifies the patient according to agency policy using two identifiers; attends appropriately to standard precautions, hand hygiene, safety, privacy, body mechanics, and documentation.			
Daily Preparation of Equipment:			
1. Prepares the equipment. An inline suction unit is available only for patients on a mechanical ventilator. Most agencies require the respiratory therapy department to set up the inline suction equipment. If this is not the agency's policy, performs the following to prepare equipment for future use. These steps need to be performed only one time per day. a. Opens the inline suction catheter using sterile technique.			
b. Removes the adapter on the ventilator tubing.			
c. Attaches the inline suction catheter equipment to the ventilator tubing.			
d. Reconnects the adapter on the ventilator tubing.			
e. Attaches the other end of the inline suction catheter to the connection tubing.			
Suctioning Procedure Steps:			
2. Positions patient in a semi-Fowler's position, unless contraindicated.			
3. Dons procedure gloves.			
4. Places linen-saver pad or towel on patient's chest.			
5. If a lock is present on the suction control port, unlocks it.			
6. Turns on the wall suction or portable suction machine and adjusts the pressure regulator according to agency policy (typically 100–150 mm Hg for adults, 95–120 mm Hg for children, and 50–95 mm Hg for infants).			
7. Uses dominant hand to pick up the catheter; uses nondominant hand for the suction port.			

PROCEDURE STEPS	Yes	No	COMMENTS
8. Unlocks the catheter and gently inserts the suction catheter into the airway by maneuvering the catheter within the sterile sleeve.			
9. Advances the suction catheter into the airway to the pre-marked distance being careful not to force the catheter.			
a. Asks patient to take slow, deep breaths.			
b. Does not force if there is resistance.			
c. Does not apply suction while advancing the catheter.			
10. Applies suction by depressing the button over the suction control port, while withdrawing the catheter. Makes sure to apply suction for no longer than 15 seconds.			
11. Withdraws the inline suction catheter completely into the sleeve. The indicator line on the catheter should appear through the sleeve.			
12. Attaches the prefilled, 10-mL container of normal saline solution to the saline port located on the inline equipment.			
13. Squeezes the 10-mL container of normal saline while applying suction.			
14. Locks the suction regulator port.			

Recommendation: Pass _____ Needs more practice _____

Student: _____   Date: _____

Instructor: _____   Date: _____

Check (✓) Yes or No

PROCEDURE STEPS	Yes	No	COMMENTS
Before, during, and after the procedure, follows Principles-Based Checklist to Use With All Procedures, including: Identifies the patient according to agency policy using two identifiers; attends appropriately to standard precautions, hand hygiene, safety, privacy, body mechanics, and documentation.			
1. Positions patient: a. For oropharyngeal suctioning: semi-Fowler's or high Fowler's position with his head turned toward the nurse			
b. Nasopharyngeal suctioning: semi-Fowler's or high-Fowler's position with his neck hyperextended (unless contraindicated)			
2. Places the linen-saver pad or towel on patient's chest.			
3. Puts on a face shield or goggles and gown.			
4. Turns on the wall suction or portable suction machine and adjusts the pressure regulator according to policy (usually 100–150 mm Hg for adults, 100–120 mm Hg for children, and 50–95 mm Hg for infants).			
5. Tests the suction equipment by occluding the connection tubing.			
6. Opens the suction catheter kit or the gathered equipment if a kit is not available. If using the nasal approach, opens the water-soluble lubricant.			
7. Dons procedure gloves; keeps the dominant hand clean; considers nondominant hand to be contaminated.			
8. Pours sterile saline into the sterile container, using the nondominant hand.			
9. Picks up the suction catheter with the dominant hand and attaches it to the connection tubing (to suction).			
10. Puts the tip of the suction catheter into the sterile container of normal saline solution and suctions a small amount of normal saline solution through the suction catheter. Applies suction by placing a finger over the suction control port.			

PROCEDURE STEPS	Yes	No	COMMENTS
11. Approximates the depth to which to insert the suction catheter: a. *Oropharyngeal suctioning*: Measures the distance between the edge of patient's mouth and the tip of patient's earlobe.			
b. *Nasopharyngeal suctioning*: Measures the distance between the tip of patient's nose and the tip of patient's earlobe.			
12. Using the nondominant hand, removes the oxygen delivery device, if present. Asks patient to take several slow, deep breaths. (It is not necessary to remove the oxygen if patient is on nasal oxygen and suctioning is via oropharynx.)			
13. If patient's oxygen saturation is less than 94%, or if he is in any distress, administers supplemental oxygen before, during, and after suctioning. See Procedure Checklist Chapter 36: Administering Oxygen (by Cannula, Face Mask, or Face Tent).			
14. Lubricates and inserts the suction catheter: a. *Oropharyngeal suctioning* 1) Lubricates the catheter tip with normal saline. 2) Using the dominant hand, gently but quickly inserts the suction catheter along the side of patient's mouth into the oropharynx. 3) Advances the suction catheter quickly to the premeasured distance (usually 7.5–10 cm [3–4 in.] in the adult), being careful not to force the catheter.			
b. *Nasopharyngeal suctioning* 1) Lubricates the catheter tip with the water-soluble lubricant. 2) Using the dominant hand, gently but quickly inserts the suction catheter into the naris. 3) Advances the suction catheter quickly to the premeasured distance (13–15 cm [5– 6 in.] in an adult), being careful not to force the catheter. 4) If resistance is met, tries using the other naris.			
15. Places a finger (thumb) over the suction control port of the suction catheter and starts suctioning patient. Applies suction while withdrawing the catheter in a continuous rotating motion.			
16. Limits suctioning to 10–15 seconds.			

PROCEDURE STEPS	Yes	No	COMMENTS
17. After the catheter is withdrawn, clears it by placing the tip of the catheter into the container of sterile saline and applying suction.			
18. Lubricates the catheter and repeats suctioning as needed, allowing at least 20-second intervals between suctioning. For nasopharyngeal suctioning, alternates nares each time suction is repeated.			
19. Coils the suction catheter in the dominant hand. Pulls the sterile glove off over the coiled catheter. (Alternatively, wraps the catheter around the dominant gloved hand and holds the catheter while removing the glove over it.)			
20. Using the nondominant hand, clears the connecting tubing of secretions by placing the tip into the container of sterile saline.			
21. Disposes of equipment in a biohazard bag.			
22. Makes sure new suction supplies are available for future suctioning.			
23. Provides mouth care.			
24. Discards other glove and remaining supplies.			
25. Positions patient comfortably and allows him to rest.			

Recommendation: Pass _____ Needs more practice _____

Student: _____   Date: _____

Instructor: _____   Date: _____

Check (✓) Yes or No

PROCEDURE STEPS	Yes	No	COMMENTS
Before, during, and after the procedure, follows Principles-Based Checklist to Use With All Procedures, including: Identifies the patient according to agency policy using two identifiers; attends appropriately to standard precautions, hand hygiene, safety, privacy, body mechanics, and documentation.			
1. Obtains and prepares the prescribed drainage system. a. *Disposable water-seal system (CDU) without suction:* 1) Removes the cover on the water-seal chamber and, using the funnel provided, fills the second (water-seal) chamber with sterile water or normal saline. Fills to the 2-cm mark, or as indicated. 2) Places the CDU upright at least 30 cm (1 ft) below patient's chest level. 3) Replaces the cover on the water-seal chamber. 4) Goes to Step 2.			
b. *Disposable water-seal CDU with suction:* 1) Removes the cover on the water-seal chamber and, using the funnel provided, fills the water-seal chamber (second chamber) with sterile water or normal saline to the 2-cm mark. 2) Adds sterile water or normal saline solution to the suction-control chamber. Adds the amount of fluid specified by the physician prescription, typically 20 cm (7 in.). 3) Places the CDU upright and at least 30 cm (1 ft) below patient's chest level. 4) Attaches the tubing from the suction-control chamber to the connecting tubing attached to the suction source. Turns on the suction; a wall suction of –80 cm H_2O is common. 5) Goes to Step 2.			
c. *Disposable dry-seal CDU with suction:* 1) Removes nonsterile outer bag and the sterile inner wrapping. 2) Places CDU upright at least 30 cm (1 ft) below patient's chest level.			

PROCEDURE STEPS	Yes	No	COMMENTS
3) If suction will be required, attaches tubing from the suction control chamber to the connecting tubing from the suction source. 4) Fills a syringe with 45 mL of sterile water or saline (follow agency policy and manufacturer's recommendations), or uses the small bottle of sterile fluid in the CDU package. Fills the air leak monitor on the CDU by injecting the fluid into the needleless injection port on the back, to the fill line. 5) Goes to Step 2.			
d. *Heimlich valve:* If there is little or no drainage and a Heimlich valve is prescribed, attaches it to the end of the chest tube when it is inserted. Goes to Step 2.			
Inserting the Chest Tube:			
2. Positions patient according to the indicated insertion site.			
3. Opens the chest tube insertion tray and sets up the sterile field. Using sterile technique, drops any necessary supplies on the field.			
4. Dons a mask, gown, and sterile gloves.			
5. Organizes the supplies that will be needed for dressing the site after insertion.			
6. Provides support to patient while the physician prepares the sterile field, anesthetizes patient, and inserts and sutures the chest tube.			
7. As soon as the chest tube is inserted, attaches it to the CDU, using a connector.			
8. If suction is prescribed, adjusts the CDU suction to the level the clinician specifies, usually -20 cm H_2O, and adjusts the wall (or other) suction source, usually to -80 cm H_2O. a. *Water-seal drainage unit:* Adjusts the suction source until gentle bubbling occurs in the suction control chamber.			
b. *Dry-seal drainage unit:* Adjusts CDU suction (e.g., to -20 cm H_2O) by turning the suction control dial on the CDU. Adjusts the wall suction pressure to -80 mm Hg or greater until the display on the suction-control chamber confirms adequate suction.			

PROCEDURE STEPS	Yes	No	COMMENTS
c. *No suction prescribed:* Leaves the suction tubing on the drainage system open. (Follows the manufacturer's directions on the CDU; models differ.)			
Dressing the Chest Tube:			
(When the chest tube is functioning properly, the physician will suture it in place.)			
9. Dons a new pair of sterile gloves.			
10. Using sterile technique, wraps petroleum gauze around the chest tube insertion site (unless the physician chooses to dress the site.)			
11. Places a precut, sterile, split-drain dressing over the petroleum gauze.			
12. Places a second sterile, precut drain dressing over the first drain dressing with the opening facing in the opposite direction from the first one.			
13. Places a large drainage dressing (ABD) over the two precut drain dressings.			
14. Secures the dressing in place (e.g., with 2-in. silk tape), making sure to cover the dressing completely.			
15. Writes date, time, and initials on the dressing.			
16. Using the spiral taping technique, wraps 1-inch silk tape around the chest tube starting above the connector and continuing below the connector. Reverses the wrapping by taping back up the tubing (using the spiral technique) until above the connector. (Or uses commercial banding gun to secure connections.)			
17. Cuts an 8-inch-long piece of 2-inch tape. Loops one end around the top portion of the drainage tube and secures the remaining end of the tape to the chest tube dressing.			
18. Makes sure that the drainage tubing lies with no kinks from the chest tube to the drainage chamber.			
19. Prepares patient for a portable chest x-ray.			
20. Places two rubber-tipped clamps at patient's bedside for special situations (safety measure).			
21. Places a petroleum gauze dressing at the bedside in case the chest tube becomes dislodged.			
22. Keeps a spare disposable drainage system at patient's bedside.			
23. Positions patient for comfort, as indicated, but with head of bed elevated to at least 30 degrees.			

PROCEDURE STEPS	Yes	No	COMMENTS
24. Maintains chest tube and drainage system patency by, for example: a. Making sure the drainage tubing is free of kinks.			
b. Inspecting the air vent in the drainage system to make sure it is patent.			
c. Making sure the drainage system is located below the insertion site.			

Recommendation: Pass _____ Needs more practice _____

Student: _____ Date: _____

Instructor: _____ Date: _____

 Copyright © 2016, F. A. Davis Company, Wilkinson & Treas/Procedure Checklists for Fundamentals of Nursing, 3e

PROCEDURE CHECKLIST
Chapter 36: Tracheostomy Care Using Sterile Technique

Check (✓) Yes or No

PROCEDURE STEPS	Yes	No	COMMENTS
Before, during, and after the procedure, follows Principles-Based Checklist to Use With All Procedures, including: Identifies the patient according to agency policy using two identifiers, attends appropriately to standard precautions, hand hygiene, safety, privacy, body mechanics, and documentation.			
1. Places patient in semi-Fowler's position.			
2. Places a towel or linen-saver pad over patient's chest.			
3. Dons sterile gloves, gown, and face shield or mask. (For modified sterile technique, dons clean procedure gloves.)			
4. Suctions the tracheostomy (see Procedure Checklist Chapter 36: Performing Tracheostomy or Endotracheal Suctioning). a. if there is a Passy-Muir valve, removes it before suctioning.			
5. Removes and discards the soiled tracheostomy dressing in a biohazard receptacle; then removes and discards gloves and performs hand hygiene.			
6. Places the tracheostomy care equipment on the overbed table and prepares the equipment using sterile technique: *Disposable inner cannula*: Pours sterile normal saline into the two sterile containers, according to agency policy. (For modified sterile technique, uses filtered tap water or sterile normal saline, per agency policy.)			
Reusable inner cannula: a. Pours hydrogen peroxide into one of the sterile solution containers and sterile saline solution into the other one.			
b. Opens two 4 in. × 4 in. gauze packages; wets the gauze in one package with sterile normal saline; keeps the second package dry. (For modified sterile technique, instead of sterile gauze, uses disposable prepackaged wipes.)			

PROCEDURE STEPS	Yes	No	COMMENTS
c. Opens one cotton-tipped applicator package. Wets the applicators with sterile saline solution (or filtered tap water or normal saline solution, for modified sterile technique).			
7. Opens the package containing a new disposable inner cannula, if available.			
8. Opens the package of Velcro tracheostomy ties or cuts a length of twill tape long enough to go around patient's neck two times. Cuts the end of the tape on an angle.			
9. Positions a biohazard bag within reach.			
10. Dons sterile gloves or a sterile glove on dominant hand and a clean glove on nondominant hand; keeps the glove on the dominant hand clean. Handles the sterile supplies with the dominant hand only. (For modified sterile technique, dons clean procedure gloves.)			
11. **For patients receiving oxygen:** With the nondominant (nonsterile) hand, removes the humidification or oxygen source. Attaches O_2 source to outer cannula if possible. a. *Reusable inner cannula*: If O_2 source cannot be attached to outer cannula, has respiratory therapist set up oxygen blow-by to use while cleaning the inner cannula.			
12. Unlocks and removes the inner cannula with the nondominant hand and cares for it accordingly: *Disposable inner cannula*: a. Disposes of the inner cannula in the biohazard receptacle according to agency policy.			
b. With the dominant hand, inserts new inner cannula into the tracheostomy in the direction of the curvature.			
c. Following manufacturer's instructions, locks the inner cannula in place.			
d. Keeps the dominant hand sterile. (For modified sterile technique, keeps dominant hand clean.)			
Reusable inner cannula: e. Places inner cannula into basin with hydrogen peroxide. Picks it up with the nonsterile hand. With sterile hand, uses the sterile nylon brush to scrub the cannula.			

PROCEDURE STEPS	Yes	No	COMMENTS
f. Immerses inner cannula in sterile normal saline (for modified sterile procedure, tap water or normal saline) and agitates it until rinsed thoroughly.			
g. Taps the inner cannula against the side of the container to remove excess saline. (For modified sterile technique, shakes the cannula to remove water.)			
h. With the dominant hand, reinserts the inner cannula into the tracheostomy, in the direction of the curvature.			
i. Following manufacturer's instructions, locks the inner cannula in place securely.			
j. Keeps the dominant hand sterile.			
13. If patient has a Passy–Muir valve (PMV), cleans it in the following manner: a. First, swishes the valve in warm filtered tap water with mild soap.			
b. Then, rinses the PMV thoroughly in warm filtered tap water.			
c. Does not use hot water, peroxide, bleach, vinegar, alcohol, brushes, or Q-tips to clean.			
d. Next, shakes the PMV to remove excess fluid.			
14. Cleans the stoma under the faceplate with cotton-tipped applicators saturated with sterile normal saline. Or uses the gauze pads, if contained in the tracheostomy kit. (Or for modified sterile technique, uses distilled or filtered tap water, or prepackaged disposable wipes.) a. Uses a circular motion from the stoma site outward.			
b. Uses each applicator only once, then discards.			
15. Cleans the top surface of faceplate and surrounding skin with gauze pads saturated with sterile normal saline solution (distilled or filtered tap water, if modified sterile technique). Uses each pad only once, then discards it.			
16. Dries the skin and outer cannular surfaces by patting them lightly with the remaining dry gauze pad.			

PROCEDURE STEPS	Yes	No	COMMENTS
17. Asks another staff member to help change tracheostomy stabilizers.			
18. Removes soiled tracheostomy stabilizers. a. *Velcro stabilizers*: With an assistant stabilizing the tracheostomy tube, disengages the soiled Velcro on both sides and gently removes from the eyes of the faceplate and discards in biohazard container.			
b. *Twill tape*: With an assistant stabilizing the trach tube, cuts soiled ties with bandage scissors. Takes care not to cut the tube of the trach balloon. Gently removes soiled ties from faceplate and discards in biohazard container.			
19. Asks patient to flex his neck or asks an assistant to hold patient's head forward (still stabilizing the tracheostomy); applies new tracheostomy stabilizers. *Velcro stabilizers* a. Threads one end of the holder through a faceplate eyelet and fastens the Velcro.			
b. Brings the holder around the back of patient's neck, threads it through the other faceplate eyelet, and fastens securely.			
c. Places one finger under the holder to check that it is secure but not too tight.			
Twill tape d. Threads one end of the tape into one of the faceplate eyelets; pulls it through and brings both ends of the tape together.			
e. Brings both ends of the twill tape around the back of patient's neck and threads them through the back of the empty faceplate eyelet.			
f. Asks the assistant to place one finger under the twill tape while tying the two ends together in a square knot.			
20. Inserts a precut, sterile tracheostomy dressing under the face plate and clean stabilizers (or folds a 4 in. × 4 in. gauze into a V-shape). Does not cut gauze.			
21. Replaces Passy–Muir valve as appropriate.			
22. Disposes of used equipment in the appropriate biohazard receptacle according to agency policy.			

 Copyright © 2016, F. A. Davis Company, Wilkinson & Treas/Procedure Checklists for Fundamentals of Nursing, 3e

PROCEDURE STEPS	Yes	No	COMMENTS

<u>Recommendation:</u> Pass _____ Needs more practice _____

Student: _____   Date: _____

Instructor: _____   Date: _____

Copyright © 2016, F. A. Davis Company, Wilkinson & Treas/Procedure Checklists for Fundamentals of Nursing, 3e

PROCEDURE CHECKLIST
Chapter 37: Performing Cardiac Monitoring

Check (✓) Yes or No

PROCEDURE STEPS	Yes	No	COMMENTS
Before, during, and after the procedure, follows Principles-Based Checklist to Use With All Procedures, including: Identifies the patient according to agency policy using two identifiers; attends appropriately to standard precautions, hand hygiene, safety, privacy, body mechanics, and documentation.			
1. a. *For hardwire monitoring*: Plugs the monitor into an electrical outlet and turns it on. Connects the cable with lead wires into the monitor.			
b. *For telemetry monitoring*: Inserts a new battery into the transmitter; turns on the transmitter; connects the lead wires to the transmitter (if not permanently attached), taking care to attach each one to its correct outlet.			
2. Exposes patient's chest and identifies electrode sites based on the monitoring system being used and patient's anatomy.			
3. Gently rubs the placement sites with a washcloth or gauze pad until the skin reddens slightly.			
4. If patient's chest contains dense hair, shaves or clips the hair with scissors at each electrode site.			
5. Cleans the areas chosen for electrode placement with an alcohol pad; allows them to dry.			
6. Removes the electrode backing and makes sure the gel is moist. Applies the electrodes to the sites by pressing firmly.			
7. Attaches the lead wires to the electrodes by snapping or clipping them in place.			
8. Secures the monitoring equipment. a. *For hardwire monitoring*: Wraps a piece of 1-in. tape around the cable and secures it to patient's gown with a safety pin.			
b. *For telemetry monitoring*: Places the transmitter in the pouch and ties the pouch strings around patient's neck and waist. Places the transmitter into patient's robe pocket if a pouch is not available.			
9. Checks patient's ECG tracing on the monitor. If necessary, adjusts the gain on the monitor to increase the waveform size.			

PROCEDURE STEPS	Yes	No	COMMENTS
10. Sets the upper and lower heart rate alarm limits according to agency policy or patient's condition and turns them on.			
11. Obtains a rhythm strip by pressing the "record" button. a. *For hardwire monitoring:* Presses the "record" button on the bedside monitor.			
b. *For telemetry monitoring:* Presses the "record" button on the transmitter of the telemetry unit.			
12. Interprets the rhythm strip and mounts it appropriately (e.g., with transparent tape) in patient's record.			

Recommendation: Pass _____ Needs more practice _____

Student: _____ Date: _____

Instructor: _____ Date: _____

Chapter 38: Assisting With Percutaneous Central Venous Catheter Placement

Check (✔) Yes or No

PROCEDURE STEPS	Yes	No	COMMENTS
Before, during, and after the procedure, follows Principles-Based Checklist to Use With All Procedures, including: Identifies the patient according to agency policy using two identifiers; attends appropriately to standard precautions, hand hygiene, safety, privacy, and body mechanics.			
1. Explains the procedure to patient.			
2. Verifies informed consent.			
3. Takes baseline vital signs.			
4. Gathers supplies and performs meticulous hand hygiene.			
5. Sets up sterile field.			
6. Positions table so it is easily accessible by the physician or advanced practice nurse (APN).			
7. Positions patient in Trendelenburg with a rolled towel between the shoulders.			
8. After the physician or APN performs hand hygiene, offers mask, gown, sterile gloves, etc.			
9. Dons mask and sterile gloves (in that order).			
10. Uses gown and maximum barrier precautions.			
11. Preps the site with approved chlorhexidine-containing antiseptic solution: a. Using back-and-forth motion, scrubs 8 × 10-in. area. Does not go back over an area with the same applicator.			
b. Repeats with three applicators, scrubbing for at least 30 seconds (2 minutes for moist site).			
c. Allows site to air-dry completely (about 2 minutes); does not touch, wipe, or blot dry.			
12. Drapes insertion site, exposing only the prepared skin. Uses other large drape (or two smaller drapes) to cover patient head to toe.			
13. If patient is not wearing a mask, instructs him to turn his head in the opposite direction of insertion.			
14. Observes while physician or APN anesthetizes the area, primes, inserts, and sutures the catheter in place.			
15. When the physician or APN is finished, applies sterile transparent dressing over the site.			
16. If there are clamps on the lumens, closes them.			

PROCEDURE STEPS	Yes	No	COMMENTS
17. Places tape over the lumens near the ends, but not on the injection caps.			
18. Removes sterile drape.			
19. Assists patient to a comfortable position.			
20. Disposes of used supplies and equipment.			
21. Removes and disposes of mask and gloves.			
22. Performs hand hygiene.			

Recommendation: Pass _____ Needs more practice _____

Student: _____   Date: _____

Instructor: _____   Date: _____

370   Copyright © 2016, F. A. Davis Company, Wilkinson & Treas/Procedure Checklists for Fundamentals of Nursing, 3e

PROCEDURE CHECKLIST
Chapter 38: Changing IV Dressings

Check (✓) Yes or No

PROCEDURE STEPS	Yes	No	COMMENTS
Before, during, and after the procedure, follows Principles-Based Checklist to Use With All Procedures, including: Identifies the patient according to agency policy using two identifiers; attends appropriately to standard precautions, hand hygiene, safety, privacy, and body mechanics.			
Changing Peripheral IV Dressing:			
1. Wearing clean nonsterile gloves, stabilizes the catheter with the nondominant hand and carefully removes the dressing and stabilization device.			
2. Inspects the insertion site for erythema, drainage, and tenderness.			
3. Removes procedure gloves and performs hand hygiene. Then dons clean nonsterile gloves.			
4. Cleanses the insertion site with an antiseptic swab: a. If using a chlorhexidine-based product (preferred), uses a back-and-forth motion and friction for at least 30 seconds.			
b. If using alcohol or 2% tincture of iodine, starts at the insertion site and works outward 2–3 inches in a circular pattern.			
5. Allows the antiseptic to dry on the skin without fanning.			
6. Performs hand hygiene and dons clean nonsterile gloves.			
7. Applies a new sterile catheter stabilization device.			
8. Covers the insertion site with a sterile semipermeable transparent dressing. a. If not already done, opens the package containing the dressing. Removes the protective backing from the dressing, making sure not to touch the sterile surface.			
b. Covers the insertion site and the hub or winged portion of the catheter with the dressing. Does not cover the connection between the IV tubing and the catheter.			
c. Gently pinches the transparent dressing around the catheter hub to secure the hub.			

PROCEDURE STEPS	Yes	No	COMMENTS
d. Smoothes the remainder of the dressing so that it adheres to the skin.			
9. Is certain the connection between the catheter and the IV tubing is secure, but does not cover the connection with tape.			
10. Secures the IV administration tubing by looping and taping the tubing to patient.			
11. Labels the dressing with the date and time of insertion, catheter size, and the date the dressing was changed and initials.			
12. Discards supplies into the appropriate receptacles.			
Changing Central Line Dressing:			
When performing the procedure, always identify patient according to agency policy, using two identifiers; and be attentive to standard precautions, hand hygiene, patient safety and privacy, body mechanics, and documentation.			
13. Obtains sterile central line dressing kit and mask for patient, if needed.			
14. Places patient in a semi-Fowler's position if tolerated; lowers the siderail, and puts the bed at a working height.			
15. Explains the procedure to patient and asks him to turn his head to the opposite side from the insertion site. If patient is unable or uncooperative, places a mask on him.			
16. Dons mask and clean nonsterile gloves and carefully removes the old dressing and catheter stabilization device if one is present. If a drape comes in the kit, applies it.			
17. Inspects the site for complications.			
18. Removes and discards gloves and soiled dressing.			
19. Performs hand hygiene.			
20. Sets up a sterile field and opens the dressing kit.			
21. Dons sterile gloves contained in the kit.			
22. Arranges sterile supplies, as needed.			

PROCEDURE STEPS	Yes	No	COMMENTS

23. Scrubs the insertion site and surrounding skin with an antiseptic swab.
   a. If using chlorhexidine-containing products (preferred), uses a back-and-forth motion and friction for at least 30 seconds.
   b. If using alcohol or 2% tincture of iodine, starts at the insertion site and works outward 2–3 inches in a circular pattern.			

24. Scrubs the catheter hubs, extension tails, any sutures, and exposed catheter with a sterile swab.			
25. Allows site to dry; does not fan.			
26. Applies a new sterile catheter stabilization device, if one is available.			

27. Applies transparent dressing that comes in the kit.
   a. *If using a folded sterile gauze* under the catheter hub, places it first.
   b. *If using a chlorhexidine gluconate sponge* as part of dressing, applies it directly over the catheter insertion site, then applies transparent dressing over all.			

28. Removes the drape, if one was used.			
29. Loops the catheter as needed and secures it with tape to the skin. Avoids securing it to the dressing. Or, depending on the type of CVC, places clear tape across the ends of the lumens near, but not on, the hubs.			
30. Labels the dressing with the date changed, time, and initials.			
31. Removes mask and gloves; removes mask from patient.			
32. Places patient in a comfortable position, raises siderail, and places call light so it is accessible.			
33. Disposes of supplies into the appropriate receptacles.			
Changing PICC Line Dressings:			
Before, during, and after the procedure, follows Principles-Based Checklist to Use With All Procedures, including: Identifies the patient according to agency policy using two identifiers; attends appropriately to standard precautions, hand hygiene, safety, privacy, and body mechanics.			
34. Obtains sterile central line dressing kit (or equivalent supplies if there is no kit) and mask for the patient, if one is needed.			

PROCEDURE STEPS	Yes	No	COMMENTS
35. Places patient in semi-Fowler's position.			
36. Explains the procedure to patient.			
37. Asks the patient to turn his head to the opposite side of the insertion site; if unable, places a mask on the patient, if consistent with agency policy.			
38. Inspects the site for signs and symptoms of infection.			
39. Dons mask and nonsterile gloves and removes old dressing, pulling toward the insertion site.			
40. Removes and discard gloves along with the old dressing.			
41. Performs hand hygiene, opens dressing change kit, and dons sterile gloves.			
42. Sets up sterile field and arranges supplies.			
43. Uses sterile tape measure to compare the external length of PICC to base insertion length, if consistent with agency's policy.			
44. Scrubs the catheter's insertion site and the surrounding area that will be covered by the dressing for 30 seconds, if using chlorhexidine, or per manufacturer's guidelines. Allows to air-dry completely.			
45. If using a chlorhexidine sponge as part of the dressing, applies directly over the insertion site; ensures that it is in direct contact with the skin.			
46. Applies the stabilization device, if applicable.			
47. Applies the transparent dressing that comes in the kit. Loops the catheter and injection camp so that it is pointing up.			
48. Labels the dressing with the date, time, and initials.			
49. Loops and anchors the catheter; secures with tape.			
50. Disposes of used supplies and equipment.			
51. Performs hand hygiene.			

Recommendation: Pass _____ Needs more practice _____

Student: _____   Date: _____

Instructor: _____   Date: _____

PROCEDURE CHECKLIST
Chapter 38: Changing IV Solutions and Tubing

Check (✓) Yes or No

PROCEDURE STEPS	Yes	No	COMMENTS
Before, during, and after the procedure, follows Principles-Based Checklist to Use With All Procedures, including: Identifies the patient according to agency policy using two identifiers; attends appropriately to standard precautions, hand hygiene, safety, privacy, and body mechanics.			
Changing the IV Solution:			
1. Using the "rights" of medication administration, prepares and labels the next container of IV solution 1 hour before the present infusion is scheduled for completion.			
2. Closes the roller clamp on the infusing administration set.			
3. Wearing clean nonsterile gloves, removes the old IV solution container from the IV pole. Removes the spike from the bag, keeping the spike sterile.			
4. Removes the protective cover from the new IV solution container port and spikes the new solution container, maintaining sterility. *For a glass IV container*, first scrubs the rubber stopper on the top of the bottle with an alcohol pad.			
5. Hangs the IV solution container on the IV pole.			
6. Inspects the tubing to be sure that it is free of air bubbles and the drip chamber is half-filled. Flicks the tubing with a finger to mobilize the bubbles into the drip chamber as needed.			
7. Opens the roller clamp and adjusts the drip rate, as prescribed (or starts infusion pump).			
8. If practiced in the agency, affixes a time tape to the new IV solution container. Marks the tape with infusion start time, and at 1-hour intervals until reaching the bottom of the container.			
9. Disposes of supplies into appropriate receptacles.			
Changing the IV Administration Tubing and Solution:			
10. Using the "rights" of medication administration, prepares and labels the next container of IV solution at least 1 hour before the present infusion is scheduled for completion.			

PROCEDURE STEPS	Yes	No	COMMENTS
11. Prepares the IV solution and tubing as though initiating a new IV. (See Procedure 38-1 in Vol. 2.)			
12. Hangs the new administration set on the IV pole.			
13. Closes the roller clamp on the old administration set.			
14. Wearing clean nonsterile gloves, places a sterile swab under the catheter hub.			
15. Applies pressure to the vein about 3 in. above the insertion site, using the fourth or fifth finger of the nondominant hand, while holding the catheter hub firmly with the thumb and finger of that hand.			
16. Does not apply downward pressure.			
17. Carefully removes the device securing the catheter-tubing connection (this may be as simple as turning a Luer-Lock). The connection should not be taped; if it is, removes tape.			
18. Removes the protective cover from the distal end of the new administration set.			
19. Continues to stabilize the IV catheter with the nondominant hand while applying pressure over the vein.			
20. Gently disengages old tubing from the IV catheter and places the end in a basin or other receptacle. Quickly inserts the new tubing into the catheter hub.			
21. Opens the roller clamp on the new administration set and allows the IV solution to infuse.			
22. Using the roller clamp, adjusts the flow until the prescribed rate is achieved. *If using a volume control pump:* Programs and turns on the pump.			
23. Cleanses the IV site and secures the IV catheter and tubing connection.			
24. Loops and tapes tubing to patient's skin.			
25. Labels tubing and solution with date, initials, rate, and time tape.			
26. Disposes of supplies into the appropriate receptacles.			

Recommendation: Pass _____ Needs more practice _____

Student: _____   Date: _____

Instructor: _____   Date: _____

PROCEDURE CHECKLIST
Chapter 38: Converting a Primary Line to a Peripheral IV Lock

Check (✓) Yes or No

PROCEDURE STEPS	Yes	No	COMMENTS
Before, during, and after the procedure, follows Principles-Based Checklist to Use With All Procedures, including: Identifies the patient according to agency policy using two identifiers; attends appropriately to standard precautions, hand hygiene, safety, privacy, and body mechanics.			
1. Gathers necessary supplies, including two filled flush syringes.			
2. Helps patient assume a comfortable position that provides access to his IV site.			
3. Lowers siderails, raises bed, and places linen-saver pad under extremity with IV.			
4. Dons clean nonsterile gloves.			
5. Removes the IV lock from the package and flushes the adapter with the first syringe of saline or dilute heparin, according to agency policy; places the lock back loosely inside the sterile package, using aseptic technique. **Variation: Primary tubing has extension tubing with a lock connected to the catheter hub:** Stops the infusion, disconnects the primary tubing from the extension tubing, flushes the extension tubing and continues to Step 14.			
6. Carefully removes the IV dressing and the tape that is securing the tubing.			
7. Closes the roller clamp on the administration set.			
8. With the side of the nondominant hand, applies pressure over the vein just above the insertion site while stabilizing the catheter hub.			
9. Gently disengages the old tubing from the IV catheter. If the tubing does not separate from the catheter, appropriately uses the hemostat.			
10. Quickly inserts the lock adapter into the IV catheter and turns the lock adapter until snug.			
11. Scrubs the injection port of the adapter with an antiseptic pad.			

PROCEDURE STEPS	Yes	No	COMMENTS
12. Inserts the second syringe with the flush into the injection port of the adapter. Flushes the catheter using turbulence and positive end-pressure technique (or the method recommended by the agency).			
13. Using aseptic technique, opens the package, removes the dressing, and covers the insertion site and the catheter hub with a sterile transparent semipermeable dressing.			
a. Covers the insertion site and the hub or winged portion of the catheter with the dressing.			
b. Does not cover the junction of the catheter hub and the IV lock.			
c. Gently pinches the transparent dressing around the catheter hub to secure the hub.			
d. Smoothes the remainder of the dressing so that it adheres to the skin.			
e. Labels dressing with date change and initials.			
14. Discards used supplies into appropriate receptacles.			

Recommendation: Pass _____ Needs more practice _____

Student: _____   Date: _____

Instructor: _____   Date: _____

 Copyright © 2016, F. A. Davis Company, Wilkinson & Treas/Procedure Checklists for Fundamentals of Nursing, 3e

PROCEDURE CHECKLIST
Chapter 38: Discontinuing an IV Line

Check (✔) Yes or No

PROCEDURE STEPS	Yes	No	COMMENTS
Before, during, and after the procedure, follows Principles-Based Checklist to Use With All Procedures, including: Identifies the patient according to agency policy using two identifiers; attends appropriately to standard precautions, hand hygiene, safety, privacy, and body mechanics.			
1. Assists the client to a comfortable position; raises bed to working height.			
2. Places linen-savor pad under extremity with IV.			
3. Dons clean nonsterile gloves.			
4. Closes the roller clamp on the administration set.			
5. Carefully removes the IV dressing, catheter stabilization device, and tape securing the tubing.			
6. If extension tubing or saline lock is present: Disconnects the administration set tubing and closes the slide clamp on the extension tubing.			
7. Scrubs the catheter–skin junction with an approved antiseptic product for at least 15 seconds.			
8. Applies a sterile 2 in. × 2 in. gauze pad above the IV insertion site; gently removes the catheter, directing it straight along the vein. Does not press down on the gauze pad while removing the catheter.			
9. Immediately applies firm pressure with the gauze pad over the insertion site. Holds pressure for 1–3 minutes, longer if bleeding persists.			
10. Replaces the soiled 2 in. × 2 in. with a sterile 2 in. × 2 in. gauze pad folded over to form a pressure dressing. Secures it with a piece of 1-in. tape or a transparent dressing.			
11. Returns bed to low position.			
12. Discards all supplies in the appropriate receptacles according to agency policy in line with CDC guidelines.			

Recommendation: Pass _____ Needs more practice _____

Student: _____   Date: _____

Instructor: _____   Date: _____

PROCEDURE CHECKLIST
Chapter 38: Initiating a Peripheral Intravenous Infusion

Check (✓) Yes or No

PROCEDURE STEPS	Yes	No	COMMENTS
Before, during, and after the procedure, follows Principles-Based Checklist to Use With All Procedures, including: Identifies the patient according to agency policy using two identifiers; attends appropriately to standard precautions, hand hygiene, safety, privacy, and body mechanics.			
Preparing the Supplies			
1. Places patient in a comfortable position and the bed at working height; supplies within reach.			
2. Prepares the intravenous solution and administration set.			
a. Follows the rights of medication administration; checks for proper solution with the prescribed additives.			
b. Checks the expiration date on the IV solution bag.			
c. Checks solution for discoloration or particulate matter.			
d. Labels the IV solution container with patient's name, date, and own initials.			
e. Places a time tape on the solution container with the prescribed infusion rate, time the infusion began, and time of completion.			
f. Takes the administration set from the package and closes the roller clamp.			
g. Labels administration tubing with date and time.			
h. Removes the protective covers from the solution container and the spike on the administration set, keeping the spike sterile. Places the spike into the port of the solution container. *Glass Bottle:* Cleans the rubber stopper on the top of the bottle with an alcohol pad, then inserts the spike through the rubber stopper.			
3. Hangs the administration set tubing. a. Ensures the tubing is clamped; hangs the IV solution container on an IV pole.			
b. Lightly compresses the drip chamber and allows it to fill up halfway.			

PROCEDURE STEPS	Yes	No	COMMENTS
4. *If there is no extension tubing*, primes the administration set tubing as follows: a. Opens the roller clamp and allows the fluid to slowly fill the tubing.			
b. When tubing is filled, closes clamp.			
5. *If using extension tubing,* primes the administration set tubing by attaching it to the end of the administration set and primes it with the rest of the IV line; or primes it separately, as follows: a. Cleanses injection port with an alcohol pad and allows to dry.			
b. Attaches flush syringe filled with normal saline to the injection port or to the non-Luer-Lock end and slowly pushes the fluid through the tubing.			
c. Leaves flush syringe attached to the extension tubing			
6. Inspects the tubing for air and appropriately removes it. Recaps end of tubing firmly.			
Performing the Venipuncture:			
7. Places a linen-saver pad under patient's arm.			
8. Places patient's arm in a dependent position.			
9. Applies a tourniquet 10–20 cm (4–8 in.) above the selected site. Palpates the radial pulse; if no pulse is present, loosens the tourniquet and reapplies it with less tension.			
10. Locates a vein for inserting the IV catheter. Selects the most distal vein on the hand or arm. Avoids using an arm or hand that contains a dialysis graft or fistula, or the affected arm of a mastectomy patient.			
11. Palpates the vein and presses it downward, making sure that it rebounds quickly. If the vein is not adequately dilated, uses alternative techniques.			
12. After selecting the vein, loosens the tourniquet.			
13. If excessive hair is present at the venipuncture site, clips it with scissors.			
14. Dons clean nonsterile gloves.			
15. Uses an appropriate IV catheter. Using aseptic technique, opens the catheter package.			
16. Gently reapplies the tourniquet and scrubs the site, using an antiseptic swab of chlorhexidine gluconate and alcohol (preferred), or 70% alcohol, using friction.			

 Copyright © 2016, F. A. Davis Company, Wilkinson & Treas/Procedure Checklists for Fundamentals of Nursing, 3e

PROCEDURE STEPS	Yes	No	COMMENTS
17. Allows the antiseptic to dry on the skin. Does not fan.			
18. Picks up the catheter and inspects tip integrity.			
19. Informs patient of the impending "stick."			
a. *Wing-tipped (butterfly):* Grasps the catheter by the wings, using the thumb and forefinger of the dominant hand—bevel up; removes protective cap from the needle.			
b. *Over-the-needle*: Grasps the catheter by the hub, using the thumb and forefinger of the dominant hand—bevel up.			
20. Using the nondominant hand, stabilizes the vein.			
21. Holding the catheter at a 30°–45° angle, pierces the skin directly over the vein.			
22. When flashback occurs, lowers catheter angle to skin level and advances catheter and stylet into the vein.			
23. While holding the catheter in place with one hand, releases the tourniquet and removes the stylet from the catheter.			
24. Quickly connects the administration set or extension tubing to IV catheter, using aseptic technique. Secures tubing to catheter by twisting Luer-Lock or other device. Does not use tape.			
25. Still stabilizing the catheter, slowly opens the roller clamp and allows the IV fluid to flush the catheter. Adjusts the flow rate according to the prescriber's order.			
26. Secures the connection between the tubing and catheter. If the set does not have a threaded (twist-on) connection, uses other clasping devices (not tape).			
Dressing the Site:			
27. Stabilizes the catheter with a manufactured catheter stabilization device, sterile tape, or sterile surgical strips. If using tape, adheres tape only to the hub and avoids skin immediately around the puncture site.			
28. Cleans the site with an antiseptic swab and allows it to dry before applying the dressing, if needed.			
a. Covers the insertion site and the hub or winged portion of the catheter with the dressing. Does not cover the tubing of the administration set.			

PROCEDURE STEPS	Yes	No	COMMENTS
b. Gently pinches the transparent dressing around the catheter hub to secure the hub.			
c. Smooths the remainder of the dressing so that it adheres to the skin.			
29. Labels the dressing with the date and time of insertion, catheter size, and initials.			
30. Secures the IV administration tubing by looping and taping the tubing to patient.			
31. Places an arm board under the joint and secures it with tape if the insertion site is located near a joint.			
32. Disposes of all supplies, including sharps, into appropriate receptacles; raises the siderail; lowers the bed; and places patient call system within reach. Washes hands.			

Recommendation: Pass _____ Needs more practice _____

Student: _____   Date: _____

Instructor: _____   Date: _____

Check (✓) Yes or No

PROCEDURE STEPS	Yes	No	COMMENTS
Before, during, and after the procedure, follows Principles-Based Checklist to Use With All Procedures, including: Identifies the patient according to agency policy using two identifiers; attends appropriately to standard precautions, hand hygiene, safety, privacy, and body mechanics.			
1. Stops the transfusion immediately if signs or symptoms of a transfusion reaction occur.			
2. Does not flush the tubing.			
3. Disconnects the administration set from the IV catheter.			
4. Calls for help.			
5. Checks vital signs and auscultates heart and breath sounds.			
6. Maintains a patent IV catheter by hanging a new infusion of normal saline solution, using new tubing.			
7. Notifies primary provider as soon as the blood has been stopped and patient has been assessed.			
8. Places the administration set and blood product container with the blood bank form attached inside a biohazard bag and sends it to the blood bank immediately.			
9. Obtains blood (in the extremity opposite the transfusion site) and urine specimens according to agency policy.			
10. Continues to monitor vital signs frequently, at least every 15 minutes.			
11. Administers medications as prescribed.			

Recommendation: Pass _____ Needs more practice _____

Student: _____   Date: _____

Instructor: _____   Date: _____

Copyright © 2016, F. A. Davis Company, Wilkinson & Treas/Procedure Checklists for Fundamentals of Nursing, 3e

PROCEDURE CHECKLIST
Chapter 38: Regulating the IV Flow Rate

Check (✓) Yes or No

PROCEDURE STEPS	Yes	No	COMMENTS
Before, during, and after the procedure, follows Principles-Based Checklist to Use With All Procedures, including: Identifies the patient according to agency policy using two identifiers; attends appropriately to standard precautions, hand hygiene, safety, privacy, and body mechanics.			
1. Uses the checks and rights of medication administration. Checks the solution to make sure that the proper IV fluid is hanging with the prescribed additives. Also verifies the infusion rate.			
2. Calculates the hourly rate if it is not specified in the order.			
3. a. Programs rate into the infusion pump.			
b. If there is no infusion pump, correctly calculates the drip rate. Verifies calculations.			
4. Applies a time tape to the IV solution container next to the volume markings (when hanging a new bag). Adequately marks the tape (with the time started, then at 1-hour intervals).			
5. Opens the roller clamp so that the IV fluid begins to flow (when hanging a new bag).			
6. Sets the rate a. Starts the infusion pump and programs the ordered rate.			
b. Alternatively, by gravity, using a watch, counts the number of drops entering the drip chamber in 1 minute, being sure to place watch next to drip chamber for accuracy. Adjusts the roller clamp until the prescribed drip rate is achieved.			
7. Monitors the infusion rate closely for the first 15 minutes after the infusion is begun; then monitors hourly.			

Recommendation: Pass _____ Needs more practice _____

Student: _____   Date: _____

Instructor: _____   Date: _____

Copyright © 2016, F. A. Davis Company, Wilkinson & Treas/Procedure Checklists for Fundamentals of Nursing, 3e

PROCEDURE CHECKLIST
Chapter 38: Setting Up and Using Volume-Control Pumps

Check (✓) Yes or No

PROCEDURE STEPS	Yes	No	COMMENTS
Before, during, and after the procedure, follows Principles-Based Checklist to Use With All Procedures, including: Identifies the patient according to agency policy using two identifiers; attends appropriately to standard precautions, hand hygiene, safety, privacy, and body mechanics.			
1. Calculates the hourly infusion rate by dividing the volume to be infused by the number of hours it is to be infused.			
2. Verifies the calculation.			
3. Attaches the IV pump to the IV pole and plugs it in to the nearest electrical outlet.			
4. Checks to be sure that the infusion pump has a safety sticker on it and that the cord and plug are intact.			
5. Takes the administration set from the package.			
6. Closes the clamp on the administration set.			
7. If a filter is required, attaches it to the end of the administration set.			
8. Removes the protective covers and spikes the port of the solution container with the administration set, without contaminating.			
9. Labels IV tubing and solution container with the date and time and places a time tape on IV solution container.			
10. Hangs the IV solution container on the IV pole.			
11. Compresses the drip chamber of the administration set and allows it to fill halfway.			
12. Places the electronic sensor on the drip chamber between the fluid level and the origin of the drop. (If there is no electronic sensor, consults the manufacturer's instructions for setup.)			
13. Primes the administration set with fluid by opening the roller clamp and allowing the fluid to flow slowly through the tubing. Recaps tubing and closes the clamp.			
14. Inspects the tubing for the air. If air bubbles remain in the tubing, flicks the tubing with a fingernail to mobilize the bubbles into the drip chamber.			

PROCEDURE STEPS	Yes	No	COMMENTS
15. Turns on the IV pump and loads the administration tubing into the pump according to the manufacturer's instructions.			
16. Programs the pump with the prescribed infusion rate (hourly rate) and the volume to be infused (usually the total amount in the IV bag).			
17. Dons clean nonsterile gloves and scrubs the injection port or needleless connector with an antiseptic pad, or other per-agency protocol, and checks the IV site for patency.			
18. Connects the administration set adapter to the IV catheter.			
19. Unclamps the administration set tubing (opens roller clamp all the way) and presses the "start" button on the pump.			
20. Ensures that all alarms are turned on and audible.			
21. Checks the pump hourly to make sure the correct volume is infused and primes the blood tubing by allowing the saline to backflow up into the blood bag drip chamber. Threads the line through the infusion pump.			
22. At the end of the shift (or at the time specified by the agency), clears the pump of the volume infused and records the volume on the I&O form.			

Recommendation: Pass _____ Needs more practice _____

Student: _____ Date: _____

Instructor: _____ Date: _____

PROCEDURE CHECKLIST
Chapter 38: Administering a Blood Transfusion

Check (✔) Yes or No

PROCEDURE STEPS	Yes	No	COMMENTS
Before, during, and after the procedure, follows Principles-Based Checklist to Use With All Procedures, including: Identifies the patient according to agency policy using two identifiers; attends appropriately to standard precautions, hand hygiene, safety, privacy, and body mechanics.			
1. Verifies that informed consent has been obtained.			
2. Verifies the prescription, noting the indication, rate of infusion, and any pretransfusion medications.			
3. Administers any pretransfusion medications as prescribed.			
4. Ensures patient has a patent IV line or lock.			
5. Obtains IV fluid containing normal saline solution and a blood administration set.			
6. Obtains infusion pump, if possible, and blood warmer, if necessary.			
7. Wears clean nonsterile gloves whenever handling blood products.			
8. Obtains the blood product from the blood bank, according to agency policy.			
9. Verifies that the blood product matches the prescription.			
10. Inspects the blood product for color, clots, and leakage.			
11. With another qualified staff member (as deemed by the institution) verifies patient and blood product identification, as follows: a. Has patient state his full name and date of birth (if he is able) and compares it to the name and date of birth located on the blood bank form and patient ID band.			
b. Compares patient name and hospital identification number on patient's ID bracelet with patient name and hospital ID number on the blood bank form attached to the blood product.			
c. Compares the unit identification number located on the blood bank form with the identification number printed on the blood product container.			

Copyright © 2016, F. A. Davis Company, Wilkinson & Treas/Procedure Checklists for Fundamentals of Nursing, 3e

PROCEDURE STEPS	Yes	No	COMMENTS
d. Compares patient's blood type on the blood bank form with the blood type on the blood product container.			
e. If all verifications are in agreement, both staff members sign the blood bank form attached to the blood product container.			
f. Documents on the blood bank form the date and time that the transfusion was begun.			
g. Makes sure that the blood bank form remains attached to the blood product container until administration is complete.			
12. Removes the blood administration set from the package and labels the tubing with the date and time.			
13. Closes all clamps on the administration set.			
14. Removes the protective covers from the normal saline solution container port and one of the spikes located on the "Y" of the blood product administration set. Places the spike into the port of the solution container.			
15. Hangs the normal saline solution container on the IV pole.			
16. Compresses the drip chamber of the administration set and allows it to fill up halfway.			
17. Primes the administration set with normal saline, then closes the roller clamp.			
18. Inspects the tubing for air. If air bubbles remain in the tubing, flicks the tubing with a fingernail to mobilize the bubbles up into the drip chamber.			
19. Gently inverts the blood product container several times. Does not shake the bag.			
20. Removes the protective covers from the administration set and the blood product port. Carefully spikes the blood product container through the port.			
21. Hangs the blood product container on the IV pole.			
22. Obtains and records patient's vital signs, including temperature, before beginning the transfusion.			
23. Using aseptic technique, attaches the distal end of the administration set to the IV catheter.			
24. Slowly opens the roller clamp closest to the blood product.			

PROCEDURE STEPS	Yes	No	COMMENTS
25. Using the roller clamp, adjusts the drip rate. Starts slowly until 50 mL have infused, and then sets to prescribed rate if no reaction occurs. ***If using volume-control infusion pump:*** Programs the rate and pushes "start."			
26. Remains with patient during the first 5 minutes and then obtains vital signs.			
27. Makes sure that patient's call bell or light is readily available and tells him to alert the nurse immediately of any signs or symptoms of a transfusion reaction, such as back pain, chills, itching, or shortness of breath.			
28. Obtains vital signs again in 15 minutes, then again in 30 minutes, and then hourly while the transfusion infuses.			
29. After the unit has infused, closes the roller clamp to the blood product container; opens the roller clamp to the normal saline solution to flush the administration set.			
30. Closes the roller clamp and disconnects the blood administration set from the IV catheter.			
31. If another unit of blood is required, the second unit can be hung with the same administration set.			
32. Discards the empty blood container and administration set in the proper receptacle according to agency policy.			

Recommendation: Pass _____ Needs more practice _____

Student: _____   Date: _____

Instructor: _____   Date: _____

Check (✔) Yes or No

PROCEDURE STEPS	Yes	No	COMMENTS
Before, during, and after the procedure, follows Principles-Based Checklist to Use With All Procedures, including: Identifies the patient according to agency policy; attends appropriately to standard precautions, hand hygiene, safety, privacy, and body mechanics.			
1. Ensures that patient lies supine for at least 15 minutes before stocking application.			

2. Measures extremity; obtains correct size stockings.
  a. Thigh-high stockings:
    1) Measures the circumference of the upper thigh at the gluteal fold.
    2) Measures the calf circumference at the widest section.
    3) Measures the distance from the gluteal fold to the base of the heel.			

b. Knee-high stockings:
    1) Measures the circumference of the calf at the widest section.
    2) Measures the distance from the base of the heel to the middle of the knee joint.			

3. Cleanses patient's legs and feet if necessary. Dries well.			
4. Lightly dusts legs and feet with talcum powder, if available, desired, appropriate for patient, and recommended by the manufacturer.			
5. Holds top cuff in dominant hand, slides nondominant arm into stocking until hand reaches stocking heel; turns stocking inside out, stopping when the heel reaches the level of the dominant hand.			
6. Grasps the heel with hand still inside the turned ("bunched") stocking and, having patient point his toes, eases the stocking onto patient's foot.			
7. Centers patient's heel in the heel of the stocking.			
8. Gradually pulls stocking up to 1–2 in. below the knee or to the gluteal fold (depending on stocking type).			
9. Checks that stocking is straight and free of wrinkles.			
10. Tugs on stocking toe to create a small space between end of toes and stocking.			

PROCEDURE STEPS	Yes	No	COMMENTS
11. Repeats procedure on the other leg.			

Recommendation: Pass _____   Needs more practice _____

Student: _____   Date: _____

Instructor: _____   Date: _____

PROCEDURE CHECKLIST
Chapter 39: Applying Sequential Compression Devices

Check (✔) Yes or No

PROCEDURE STEPS	Yes	No	COMMENTS
Before, during, and after the procedure, follows Principles-Based Checklist to Use With All Procedures, including: Identifies the patient according to agency policy; attends appropriately to standard precautions, hand hygiene, safety, privacy, and body mechanics.			
1. Cleanses patient's legs and feet, if necessary.			
2. Applies elastic stockings if they are ordered in conjunction with the sequential pressure device (SCD).			
3. Measures extremity following manufacturer's instructions; obtains proper size sleeve.			
4. Places patient supine for at least 15 minutes before applying.			
5. Places SCD pump in a safe location near an electrical outlet and plugs it in.			
6. Applies compression sleeve correctly: a. For "Flowtron" brand sleeves (knee-length only): 1) Opens the Velcro fasteners on the sleeve. 2) Places the sleeve under the lower leg below the knee, with the "air bladder" side down on the bed. 3) Brings the ends of the sleeve up and wraps around the lower leg, leaving one to two fingerbreadths of space between the leg and the sleeve.			
b. For SCDS/PAS brand sleeves: 1) Opens Velcro fasteners on the sleeve and places the sleeve under the leg, ensuring that the fastener will close on the anterior surface. 2) For thigh-high sleeves: Places the opened sleeve under the leg, ensuring that the knee opening is at the level of the knee joint. 3) Brings the ends of the sleeve up and wraps around the lower leg, leaving one to two fingerbreadths of space between the leg and the sleeve. Wraps upper leg similarly.			
7. Connects sleeve to compression pump.			
8. Turns pump on.			
9. Sets compression pressure, if applicable, to manufacturer's recommended setting.			

PROCEDURE STEPS	Yes	No	COMMENTS

Recommendation: Pass _____   Needs more practice _____

Student: _____   Date: _____

Instructor: _____   Date: _____

PROCEDURE CHECKLIST
Chapter 39: Managing Gastric Suction

Check (✓) Yes or No

PROCEDURE STEPS	Yes	No	COMMENTS
Before, during, and after the procedure, follows Principles-Based Checklist to Use With All Procedures, including: Identifies the patient according to agency policy; attends appropriately to standard precautions, hand hygiene, safety, privacy, and body mechanics.			
Initial Equipment Setup:			
1. Places the collection container in the holder. Plugs power cord into a grounded outlet if using portable suction.			
2. Connects the short tubing between the container and the suction source ("vacuum").			
3. Connects the long suction tubing to the container. If available, connects a stopcock to the open end nearest patient.			
4. Dons clean nonsterile gloves.			
5. After nasogastric (NG) tube is inserted and placement verified, attaches the end of the NG tube to the suction tubing.			
6. If using a Salem sump tube, instills 10–20 mL of air into the vent lumen.			
7. Secures NG tube to the client's nose and to the gown.			
8. Turns on suction source to prescribed amount.			
9. Opens stopcock (if one is used).			
10. Observes that drainage appears in the collection container.			
Emptying the Suction Container:			
1. Dons clean nonsterile gloves.			
2. Turns off suction source.			
3. Closes stopcock on the tubing, or clamps tubing.			
4. Notes color, odor, and amount of drainage. If the suction canister is not marked for measuring, removes cap from the lid of the suction container and pours drainage into a graduated container to measure the amount.			
5. Empties and washes the graduated container or the suction canister.			
6. Wipes the port of the suction canister with an alcohol wipe, places the container in the holder, and closes the stopper on the port.			
7. Turns on suction source to prescribed amount; turns on the stopcock or unclamps tubing.			

PROCEDURE STEPS	Yes	No	COMMENTS
8. Observes for proper functioning of the suction and for patency of the tubing.			
9. Removes and discards gloves; performs hand hygiene.			
Irrigating the Nasogastric Tubing:			
1. Places a linen-saver pad under the NG tube.			
2. Opens the irrigation set and pours saline into the basin.			
3. Places patient at a 30°–45° elevation (unless contraindicated or not tolerated).			
4. Dons clean nonsterile gloves.			
5. Checks for correct placement of the NG tube.			
6. Fills the syringe with 10–20 mL of saline and places it on the linen-saver pad.			
7 Clamps the NG tube or turns off the stopcock. Disconnects the NG tube from the suction tubing.			
8. Holds the drainage tubing up until suction clears it, then lays it on the linen-saver pad or hooks it over the suction machine.			
9. Turns off suction machine.			
10. Unclamps the NG tube or turns on the stopcock.			
11. Unpins the NG tube (or removes tape) from patient's clothing.			
12. Attaches the syringe and instills the irrigant slowly into the NG tube. a. Does not force the solution.			
b. Does not instill fluid into the air vent.			
13. Lowers the end of the NG tube and withdraws fluid. Instills and withdraws until fluid flows freely in and out. a. *If using a double-lumen NG tube*, injects 30 mL of air into the "pigtail."			
14. Reclamps the NG tube or turns off the stopcock.			
15. Reconnects the NG tube to the suction tube; releases clamp or turns on the stopcock.			
16. Reattaches the NG tube to patient's clothing with pin or tape.			
17. Provides comfort measures (e.g., mouth care).			
18. Removes and discards gloves; performs hand hygiene.			
Providing Comfort Measures:			
1. Dons clean nonsterile gloves (unless done in conjunction with tube irrigation, preceding).			
2. Provides mouth care and mouthwash as desired; does not use lemon-glycerin swabs.			

PROCEDURE STEPS	Yes	No	COMMENTS
3. Applies water-soluble lubricant if lips are dry or crusty.			
4. Removes nasal secretions with a tissue or damp cloth.			
5. Uses a moist cotton-tip applicator to cleanse inside each nostril. If secretions are encrusted, uses hydrogen peroxide followed with water.			
6. Applies water-soluble lubricant inside each nostril.			
7. Checks that tape or tube fixation device is secure. If it is not, replaces it.			

Recommendation: Pass _____ Needs more practice _____

Student: _____   Date: _____

Instructor: _____   Date: _____

Copyright © 2016, F. A. Davis Company, Wilkinson & Treas/Procedure Checklists for Fundamentals of Nursing, 3e

PROCEDURE CHECKLIST
Chapter 39: Teaching a Patient to Deep-Breathe, Cough, Move in Bed, and Perform Leg Exercises

Check (✓) Yes or No

PROCEDURE STEPS	Yes	No	COMMENTS
Before, during, and after the procedure, follows Principles-Based Checklist to Use With All Procedures, including: Identifies the patient according to agency policy; attends appropriately to standard precautions, hand hygiene, safety, privacy, and body mechanics.			
Teaching a Patient to Deep-Breathe and Cough:			
1. Assists patient to assume Fowler's or semi-Fowler's position.			
2. For a patient with chest or abdominal incision, demonstrates splinting with blanket or pillow.			
3. *Diaphragmatic breathing*: Tells patient to: a. Place hands anteriorly along lower rib cage, third fingers touching at midline.			
b. Take deep breath slowly through the nose, feeling the chest expand.			
c. Hold her breath for 2–5 seconds, then exhale slowly and completely through the mouth.			
4. *Coughing*. Tells patient to: a. Complete two or three cycles of diaphragmatic breathing.			
b. On the next breath, lean forward and cough several times through an open mouth.			
c. If patient is too weak to cough, instructs patient to inhale deeply and perform three or four huffs against an open glottis.			
Teaching a Patient to Move in Bed:			
1. Positions patient supine, bedrails up.			
2. Instructs patient to (when turning left): a. Bend right leg, sliding foot flat along the bed and flexing knee.			
b. Reach right arm across the chest and grab the opposite bedrail.			
c. Take a deep breath, splinting any abdominal or chest incisions.			
d. Pull on the bedrail while pushing off with right foot.			
3. If patient cannot maintain position independently, places pillow or blanket along back for support.			

PROCEDURE STEPS	Yes	No	COMMENTS
Teaching Patient Leg Exercises:			
1. Positions patient supine (preferred) or in a chair.			
2. Ankle circles. Instructs patient to: a. Start with one foot in the dorsiflexed position.			
b. Slowly rotate the ankle clockwise.			
c. After three rotations, repeat the procedure in a counterclockwise direction.			
d. Repeat this exercise at least three times in each direction, then switch and exercise the other ankle.			
3. Ankle pumps. Instructs patient to: a. With leg extended, point the toe until her foot is plantar flexed.			
b. Pull the toes back toward her head until the foot is dorsiflexed; at the same time, press the back of the knee into the bed.			
c. Make sure she feels a "pull" in the calf.			
d. Repeat the alternate plantar and dorsiflexion several times.			
e. Repeat the cycle with the other foot.			
4. Leg exercises. Instructs patient to: a. Slowly begin bending the knee, sliding the sole of the foot along the bed until the knee is in a flexed position.			
b. Reverse the motion, extending the knee until the leg is once again flat on the bed.			
c. Repeat several times.			
d. Repeat using the opposite leg.			

Recommendation: Pass _____ Needs more practice _____

Student: _____   Date: _____

Instructor: _____   Date: _____

 Copyright © 2016, F. A. Davis Company, Wilkinson & Treas/Procedure Checklists for Fundamentals of Nursing, 3e